LEISURE PROGRAMS FOR HANDICAPPED PERSONS

LEISURE PROGRAMS FOR HANDICAPPED PERSONS

By

Paul Wehman, Ph.D.
Associate Professor
School of Education
Virginia Commonwealth University
Richmond, Virginia

and

Stuart J. Schleien, M.Ed.
Department of Recreation
University of Maryland
College Park, Maryland

With a contribution by **Ronald P. Reynolds**

University Park Press
Baltimore

UNIVERSITY PARK PRESS
International Publishers in Science, Medicine, and Education
300 North Charles Street
Baltimore, Maryland 21201

Copyright © 1981 by University Park Press

Typeset by Maryland Composition Company
Manufactured in the United States of America by the Maple Press Company

All rights, including that of translation into other languages, reserved. Photomechanical reproduction (photocopy, microcopy) of this book or parts thereof without special permission of the publisher is prohibited.

This publication was supported in part by a grant to Virginia Commonwealth University from Virginia State Developmental Disabilities Office (Grant Number 79-14). The Department of Mental Health and Mental Retardation reserves a royalty-free, non-exclusive, and irrevocable license to reproduce, publish, or otherwise use, and to authorize others to use, all copyrightable or copyrighted material resulting from this grant supported research.

Library of Congress Cataloging in Publication Data

Wehman, Paul.
Leisure programs for handicapped persons.

Includes index.
1. Handicapped—Recreation.   2. Leisure—Study and teaching.   3. Handicapped—Recreation—Curriculum.
I. Schleien, Stuart J., joint author.   II. Title.
GV183.5.W43   790.1'96   80-28721
ISBN 0-8391-1643-8

Contents

Preface	ix
Acknowledgments	xi

Chapter 1
NORMALIZATION
A Guideline to Leisure Skills Programming for Handicapped Individuals *Ronald P. Reynolds* 1
    The Principle: A New Direction in Human Service 1
    *The Relationship Between Normalization and Leisure 6
    Emerging Roles of Leisure Education Specialists 9

Chapter 2
LEISURE SKILLS ASSESSMENT 15
    Evaluating Leisure Skills Assessment Guides 15
    Behavioral Variables for Leisure Assessment 19
    A Model for Selection of Leisure Skills 26
    Summary 33

Chapter 3
LEISURE INSTRUCTION 37
    Program Development: Writing Behavioral Objectives ... 37
    Program Development: Task Analysis and Skill Sequencing 39
    The Need for Task Analysis Competencies 40
    Methods of Generating Skill Sequences 42
    Program Development: Teaching Techniques 45
    Program Development: Skill Generalization and Maintenance 51
    Program Development: Trainer Competencies 53
    The Final Step: Behavioral Evaluation of the Program .. 55

Chapter 4
ADAPTING LEISURE SKILLS 59
    * Rationale 59
    Historical Background 60
    Programmatic Adaptations 65
    Types of Recreational Adaptations 67
    Summary and Recommendations 85

Chapter 5
CURRICULUM DESIGN AND FORMAT 89
    Activity Groupings: Description and Rationale 89
    Skill Sequencing 92
    Core Skills 93
    Field Testing 95

Chapter 6
- **HOBBIES** 97
  - Books and Magazines 98
  - Camping 100
  - Cooking 102
  - Cycling 104
  - Holiday Activity 106
  - Musical/Rhythmical Instruments 108
  - Pet Care 110
  - Photography 113
  - Plant Care 116
  - Spectator Leisure/Community Events 118
  - Spectator Leisure/Home 119
  - Sunbathing 121
  - Table Game Hobbies 123

Chapter 7
- **SPORTS** 129
  - Badminton 130
  - Basketball 133
  - Bowling 135
  - Fishing 138
  - Handball 141
  - Jogging 143
  - Playground Equipment 144
  - Shuffleboard 148
  - Softball 149
  - Swimming 152
  - Volleyball 155
  - Weightlifting 157
  - Winter Sports 158

Chapter 8
- **GAMES** 161
  - Board and Table Games 162
  - Motor Games 172
  - Musical/Rhythmical Games 184
  - Card Games 190

Chapter 9
- **OBJECT MANIPULATION** 197
  - Blocks 198
  - Bucket and Shovel 200
  - Busy Box 202
  - Crayons 205
  - Frisbee 205

Handgripper	207
Hula-Hoop	207
Jack-in-the-Box	210
Marbles	212
Mr. Bubble	214
Multipurpose Ball	215
Scissors	218
Slinky	220
Telephone	222
Vending Machine	227

Chapter 10
PROGRAM IMPLEMENTATION
Illustrations of Recreational Competence	231
Case Study I: Teaching the Use of a Camera to a Multiply Handicapped Woman	231
Case Study II: Developing Independent Cooking Skills in a Profoundly Retarded Woman	237
Case Study III: Group Home Leisure Programming	244
Case Study IV: Teaching Multihandicapped Adults Dart Skills	252
Conclusion	259
Index	261

Preface

Within the past 5 years leisure and recreation services for handicapped individuals have received increased attention. The passage of Public Law 94–142 (Education for All Handicapped Children Act) supports therapeutic recreation as a "related service" for all handicapped students. The recently published federal regulation for rehabilitation services (Federal Register, November 1979) indicate the need for increased recreation programs for severely handicapped individuals. Several states (e.g., Virginia) have identified in their State Developmental Disabilities Plan that recreation is a priority service area for severely disabled people.

These positive developments should not come as a surprise. Since more disabled individuals than ever before are being deinstitutionalized and are returning to their respective communities, it is necessary for these persons to have appropriate social skills for community adjustment. Many of the older, previously institutionalized individuals will go to nursing homes where activity therapy is a major aspect of the daily routine. Those younger adults or children living at home will be less of a burden to the family if they are able to independently engage in leisure activity. Respite care centers are slowly being developed in communities for the purpose of short-term care for handicapped children whose parents leave on vacation or for other reasons. Staff in these centers need expertise in therapeutic recreation programming. For the more severely mentally disabled, who are still in institutions, leisure skill development is a positive means of reducing inappropriate self-stimulation or stereotypic activity.

The purpose of this book is to describe how to develop and implement leisure skill and habilitation programs for disabled individuals. Keeping with recent trends, there is a distinct emphasis on the more severely disabled. We offer assessment guidelines, instructional techniques, and special adaptations for the design of recreation programs. Curriculum material is also available in hobbies, sports, games, and object manipulation. A major objective of this book is to encourage participation and avoid exclusive reliance on sedentary leisure, a form of recreation most characteristic of handicapped individuals.

The chapters in this text have been developed in such a way as to be useful to professionals who work across numerous disability categories with individuals of all ages. There are, however, several attributes of *Leisure Programs for Handicapped Persons* that run through all aspects of the book. These attributes are:

1. A philosophy that reflects normalization theory and chronological age appropriateness in selection of leisure skills for training
2. A philosophy that supports integration of handicapped with nonhandicapped individuals
3. A philosophy that calls for the opportunity for all handicapped individuals to participate
4. A commitment to a behavior modification/learning theory–based approach to leisure training
5. A commitment to task analysis and behavioral objectives
6. A commitment to the collection of data in support of leisure training programs
7. The need for *instruction* in leisure education and generalization training *into real world community environments*
8. The need for independent use of community–based recreational facilities.

This book is intended for use by undergraduate and graduate students training in special education, recreation, and occupational therapy. It will be used by recreation therapists, special education teachers, curriculum specialists, educational administrators, occupational therapists, adult activity center staff, group home and supervised apartment staff, respite care staff, preschool teachers, and parents. All programs have been field-tested, many have been validated. The final chapter describes several data–based examples of how to develop and implement a recreation program.

Acknowledgments

We would like to express our appreciation to a number of individuals who helped us develop this textbook. We are grateful to the administrators and teachers of the greater Richmond area public schools for their assistance and encouragement.

Appreciation is also expressed to the following professionals in the field of therapeutic recreation, special education, and occupational therapy, whose valuable input through dialogue and written critiques has enabled us to develop the material: Mike Fehl, Carol Granger, Dana Guarino, Dee Dee Hill, Glenda Horst, Patti Lanier, Jo Ann Marchant, Sally Thomas, and Linda Veldheer. Their concern that this book be a valuable and convenient tool for recreators, educators, instructors, and parents has guided us throughout the course of the project.

A special thanks is also extended to Henrico County Mental Retardation Services, particularly Peggy Gould, Director, and Terri Ash, Beatrice Bullock and Meredith Minier, Instructors of the Henrico Adult Development Center, for their leisure programming assistance and support.

A word of gratitude is due to Liz Brown, Jeanne Haston, Charlotte Parks, Pat Pleasant, and Gail Worden who have labored numerous hours typing and organizing the manuscript. Their cheerful and thorough work has made our work easier.

P. W.
S. J. S.

This book is dedicated to our parents

*Helen and George Wehman
Roselyn and Herman Schleien*

LEISURE PROGRAMS FOR HANDICAPPED PERSONS

Chapter 1
NORMALIZATION
A Guideline to Leisure Skills Programming for Handicapped Individuals

Ronald P. Reynolds

THE PRINCIPLE: A NEW DIRECTION IN HUMAN SERVICE
    A recent study for the Carnegie Council on Children condemns the psychology–medicine–special education community for contributing to the damaging misconception that the handicapped are "sick" thus offering "a rationalization for excluding them from normal life."

    Associations supporting the legal rights of disabled persons assume assertive advocacy postures and lobby for "generic services" for their clientele.

    The federal government, through various funding agencies, supports personnel training demonstration projects and other efforts designed to facilitate the inclusion of disabled persons in community-based leisure settings.

    Colleges and universities reorient professional curricula to emphasize course work and practicum experiences relating to the involvement of handicapped children and adults in public education, employment, and leisure service agencies.

    Curriculum materials and journals devote increasing attention to the process of "mainstreaming."

These trends, and other related events, signal the growing commitment of human services personnel to accept and embrace the principle of normalization and utilize this philosophy as a guiding force in their interactions with handicapped individuals. Recreators and special education personnel, as well as others involved in day-to-day provision of service to disabled persons, will be profoundly influenced by this orientation in the next decade. The comprehensive and pervasive principle of normalization has dramatic implications that will alter both the content and context of leisure and educational services. Its impact will extend to and effect the very roles, techniques, and approaches we adopt toward the recreative life-styles of persons currently devalued by society. In the face of this challenge, contemporary orientations and models for the delivery of recreation and leisure services will shift markedly. Before examining the ramifications of this principle in leisure service settings, it is necessary to provide a basic insight into the origin and definition of normalization as well as a summary of existing philosophical, empirical, and legislative support for this principle.

Historical Perspective

The newness, scope, and complexity of the normalization concept have resulted in this term being frequently misunderstood, misinterpreted, and therefore regarded with suspicion in the fields of education and recreation. Much of this confusion and subsequent resistance has been due to a tendency to oversimplify the concept of normalization by equating it directly with one or a small number of its tenets. As Gunn and Peterson (1978) point out, terms such as *normalization, mainstreaming,* and *integration* are frequently used interchangeably without distinction, or without reference to the subtle but meaningful differences between these concepts. To avoid misunderstanding concerning the application of this principle in leisure services for disabled persons, it is necessary to return to a classic definition of the notion as extended by one of its leading champions and interpreters, Wolf Wolfensberger. According to this author, normalization may be viewed as:

> The utilization of means which are as culturally normative as possible, in order to establish or maintain personal behaviors or characteristics which are as culturally normative as possible (Wolfensberger, 1979, p. 28).

Extrapolating this concept to the leisure life-style of disabled persons, the following example is given to illustrate how normalization is interpreted in this realm of human experience:

> The normalization principle means making available to the mentally retarded, patterns and conditions of everyday life which are as close as possible to the norms and patterns of the mainstream of society. The normalization principle also implies a normal routine of life . . . , leisure time activities, in a variety of places (Kugel & Wolfensberger, 1969, p. 92).

With this idea concerning the application of normalization to recreation for the disabled firmly fixed, a more accurate perception regarding certain procedures prevalent in the field of leisure education may be made. For example, mainstreaming or "the educational arrangement of placing students in regular classes with their nonhandicapped peers to the maximum extent appropriate" (Turnbull & Schulz, 1979, p. 52) for the purpose of teaching leisure skills, may be thought of as one important step in the total process of normalization. Similarly, in recreational or leisure settings, the physical involvement of disabled and nondisabled persons may be construed as one objective toward achieving the goal of normalization. Conceptualizing normalization as both a *process* and a *goal*, as previously noted, has pronounced implications for those concerned with the leisure life-styles of disabled persons. This concern will extend beyond individual techniques and programs to the leisure and educational agencies and delivery systems which ultimately influence the provision of services. As Hayes (1978, p. 9) notes:

> The problems inherent in mainstreaming are not only the problems of education, physical education and/or recreation . . . they are also the problems of society at large. They are the problems of humanity.

This humanitarian concern for normalization has been bolstered by at least three areas of support that are of particular interest and relevance to recreational and educational personnel. For purposes of discussion these major areas may be classified into the categories of philosophical, empirical, and legislative influence.

Philosophical Support:
The Movement Toward Decentralization and Deinstitutionalization

The emphasis on ensuring normative patterns and conditions of life for severely developmentally disabled persons has prompted a nationwide concerted effort to develop community-based services in lieu of mass residential care. Consequently, this trend has resulted in a sharp decrease in the number of persons who will receive recreation and leisure education services within the confines of the institutional setting. As education and leisure services continue to expand in small group homes and other types of transitional living arrangements, the format and content of these programs must reflect the needs of recently discharged clients.

Pomeroy (1974) identifies the leisure and educational requirements of deinstitutionalized individuals as the development of social and self-help skills, emotional maturity, and physical mobility. As these skills are achieved by persons residing in sheltered environments in community settings, sequential processes that move persons progressively to independent leisure functioning must be implemented. Fortunately, several sound developmental models exist within the recreation/education literature to facilitate this transition. While these models differ in the variables chosen as components, each represents a powerful schema for providing a progressive continuum of service culminating in normalized recreation activity.

The first of the models, developed by Forness (1977), is designed to facilitate the transition of handicapped children from special to regular classes. Based on four stages of educational tasks, this paradigm outlines the curriculum materials, modalities, settings, reinforcers, and consequences necessary to move children through hierarchical orders of classroom settings.

A second criterion-referenced continuum for involving disabled persons in public recreation settings has been validated for use by Burdette and Miller (1979). Based in a municipal recreation facility, level one of this program is comprised of children who lack sensory motor or self-help skills. The emphasis at this level is placed on individual assessment and the upgrading of these skills. Level two deals with the development of fine and gross motor skills and activities requiring a minimum of socialization ability. Programming at the third level consists of instruction in skill-specific activities associated with sports and games. Attempts to integrate disabled and nondisabled children are made at each stage with consultant, liaison, and advocate services the primary content of the final level.

Another conceptual approach stressing a continuum of recreation programs leading to normalized participation is proposed by Hutchison and Lord (1979). These authors view the various settings in which recreation services occur as a progressive and sequential procedure. Steps in this process include: upgrading experiences in institutions, segregated upgrading experiences in associations, separate upgrading experiences in community settings, homebound and individualized programs in communities, integrated experiences in public programs with advocate support, integrated community involvement with decreased advocacy and ongoing or independent community participation.

Building upon this concept of advocacy, Stensrud (1978) outlines a strategy designed to systematically involve disabled individuals in settings requiring progressively increasing degrees of socialization. Throughout this process, with the use of volunteer assistance, procedures are utilized beginning with the inclusion of nondisabled persons in segregated settings and progressing through the stage of "50-50" (disabled/nondisabled) integration that ends in fully involved client-directed participation.

These and other models of integrated recreation programming are currently being implemented in many settings in North America. Organizations such as the Scouts, 4-H, YM-YWCAs, and service clubs are beginning to include disabled persons in regular leisure time programs instead of providing separately run facilities and opportunities for them. When properly planned and conducted, such programs can be operated less expensively than duplicate services and can contribute positively to the happiness and dignity of both disabled and nondisabled participants. For example, Braaten (1977) and Hensley (1979) provide excellent examples of guidelines that facilitate the inclusion of mentally retarded individuals in regular residential camps.

Normalization and Leisure: Emerging Empirical Support

Because of the relative newness of the normalization principle, there has been limited opportunity to systematically investigate the efficacy of this concept as applied to the leisure needs of disabled persons. Nevertheless, empirical research is beginning to emerge in recreation and special education literature that shows the potential that normalized recreation programs may have for improving the recreative functioning of handicapped persons. Similarly, the physical and social environmental conditions that affect the acceptance of disabled persons in various play settings are in the process of being delineated. To illustrate, a recent review of recreation studies spanning the period 1966 through 1975 (Matthews, 1977) isolated several instances in which the leisure involvement of handicapped and nonhandicapped children and adults resulted in improved ability of the handicapped to: 1) take part in competitive and noncompetitive games; 2) learn competencies resulting in the opportunity to return to the community; 3) participate in age–appropriate sports; 4) make gains in motor coordination and dexterity, elevate recreative functioning on selected tasks; and 5) increase purposive organized and specialized free play. In special education settings, recent investigations support the notion that planned programs of classroom integration may result in: 1) improved teacher attitudes toward disabled children and willingness to revise or adapt curricula or instructional techniques to serve these children (Harasymiw and Horne, 1975); 2) appropriate use of language and social play skills (Guralnick, 1976); and 3) a general acceptance of handicapped by nonhandicapped children in free play settings (Peterson & Haralick, 1977).

While the amount of experimental research in the recreation/education normalization literature appears to be steadily increasing, rigorous and systematic investigations into this phenomenon must continue. Variables of special interest to practitioners of leisure education curricula might include the interactive effects on the acceptance of handicapped participants by their peers of age, sex, type of disability, play environment, size and composition of the play group cohort, type and characteristics of play materials, and functional level of the participant.

Legislative Mandate

Over the past several years, there have been significant national legislative efforts designed to ensure that disabled individuals have the opportunity to function as independent members of society. Three of these legislative acts are particularly relevant to the accessibility of leisure opportunities for handicapped persons. PL 90–480 (The Architectural Barriers Act) mandates that facilities constructed after 1968 with federal monies be architecturally accessible to the disabled. The Rehabilitation Act of 1973 as amended in 1978 stresses both environmental and programmatic availability of educational and employment services. Finally, PL 94–142 (The Education for All Handicapped Children Act of 1975) has particularly far-reaching effects for providers and recipients of recreational/educational services to disabled children and young adults. Szymanski (1976) summarizes the four central purposes of this law as follows:

1. To ensure that all handicapped children have available to them special educational and related services designed to meet their unique needs (related services to include recreation)
2. To ensure that the rights of handicapped children and their parents or guardians are protected
3. To assist states and localities in providing for the education of handicapped children
4. To assess and ensure the effectiveness of efforts to educate handicapped children

Central to achieving these goals is the mandate that a written statement of specific educational services, or an individualized education program (IEP), be provided for each handicapped child. Furthermore, mainstreaming or placement of children in the "least restrictive environment" possible is emphasized.

THE RELATIONSHIP BETWEEN NORMALIZATION AND LEISURE

With the philosophical, empirical, and legislative impetus for normalization delineated, the following discussion provides an overview of the principle's major premise and corollaries, some common misconceptions concerning its implementation, and the overall concern of this text for the normalization ideology. Several of these concepts have been identified in previous works of this author (Reynolds, 1979).

1. Normalization is a multifaceted process designed to involve handicapped people in everyday life experiences (including leisure) to the maximum extent possible.

Consequently, adherence to the principle involves a variety of practices designed to reduce both the "differentness" in appearance and performance of disabled persons while simultaneously expanding the public's degree of acceptance for differentness. Key responsibilities for leisure education service providers include utilizing "culturally normative" techniques with clients which facilitate acceptance on the part of the public with whom the client will be interacting. For example, recent techniques by Wehman and Schleien (1980) involving recreational adaptations including material, skill sequence, procedural, and facility modifications have enabled severely disabled adults to participate in such normative leisure activities as bowling and photography. Such interventions have the combined effects of developing leisure skills which may generalize to other community settings and enabling the general public to observe developmentally disabled persons participating *successfully* in normal leisure pursuits.

2. The integration process, which stresses the interaction of disabled with nondisabled individuals in natural environments of everyday living, is an important corollary of normalization and as such is applicable to a wide range of disabilities.

While originally developed in conjunction with human services in the field of mental retardation, normalization has been found to be a sound principle for guiding the interactions of a variety of persons with special needs. Leisure services for visually impaired and hearing impaired individuals, for the aged, and for those with a wide variety of developmental disabilities are currently undergoing examination in order to assess their adherence to this principle. Consequently, the procedures in this text, which stress behavioral programming techniques, are applicable to many clients needing leisure skills enhancement.

3. Being "integrated" in certain leisure settings does not preclude involvement in "special" or separate programs.

Because normalization can be perceived as both a process and goal, segregated recreation programs may play an initial role in the reinvolvement of previously institutionalized clients in community-based recreation. However, special programs, catering only to disabled individuals, should be viewed as "stepping stones" to mainstream participation. For example, depending on the functional ability and needs of a developmentally disabled child, the child could be involved simultaneously in a public school curriculum designed to assess leisure preference and develop age-appropriate leisure skills, a program of remedial fine and gross motor activities provided by a local advocate association, and take part in a Saturday afternoon model building activity sponsored by the local Y. In this scenario, separate programs in schools and special interest agencies would be viewed as important efforts in sustaining and improving the child's participation in community-based opportunities. It should be noted that the assessment, leisure instruction, adaptations, materials, and curriculum presented in this text are amenable for use in a variety of recreational settings and can contribute strongly to such integrative efforts.

4. Successful integration in recreational settings depends on the involvement of small groups or individuals in existing programs or services.

Central to this principle is the notion that disabled people will be accepted more readily by their nondisabled counterparts if their numbers in a particular setting do not exceed a proportion that could reasonably be expected to occur through normal interactions. Special camps, large numbers of mentally retarded persons occupying several blocks of bowling lanes, and the inclusion of masses of disabled individuals in swimming pools illustrate the negative effect that such practices may have in leisure settings. The conceptual framework of this text, emphasizing individualized curriculum, instruction, and planned systematic leisure participation of disabled persons, is a conscious effort to avoid this barrier to achieving normalization.

5. Integration does not mean grouping people with different disabilities together.

Successful involvement of disabled persons with nondisabled individuals, not those of other disability groups, is the ultimate goal of the normalization process. Therefore, instructional or purely recreative pursuits such as handicapped horseback riding programs, special event days catering exclusively to disabled members of a community, and leagues and tournaments for handicapped participants do not achieve the ultimate goal of providing normative recreational environments. As in the previous principle, this text is concerned with the development of leisure skills and abilities which will be ultimately under the control of the individual client. The activities and skills provided and analyzed are of a small group or individual nature and intentionally do not serve as mass diversional pursuits for large groups of disabled individuals.

6. The integration process requires planning; it is not synonymous with "dumping."

As previously stated, the normalization process is comprised of a number of critical components designed to ensure that disabled persons are assimilated socially as well as physically into the mainstream of society. Therefore, meaningful involvement in leisure settings demands that attention be paid to various barriers that may prevent the inclusion of disabled persons in community-based programs. Attitudes of other staff and participants, transportation, lack of volunteer assistance, and building accessibility must be considered thoroughly and addressed in conjunction with efforts designed to upgrade the skill level of disabled persons. Readers of this text are encouraged to include these factors in any plan designed to facilitate independent leisure functioning.

7. Integration implies involvement in appropriate activities in community-based services.

The techniques and procedures described in this text may be implemented directly with disabled persons in community leisure service settings in many instances. In situations where severely handicapped individuals reside in transitional or group home facilities, the leisure skills curriculum suggested in this text stresses processes that will lead to independent leisure functioning. Specifically, leisure activities are presented that are consistent with a range of chronological ages and interests of disabled individuals. Similarly, leisure skills instruction should be conducted in settings and time frames typical of society at large. Also related to the concept of appropriate recreation is the motivation underlying participation. Because the ultimate impetus for leisure activity should be intrinsic to the individual, the leisure skills instructional techniques presented here are designed to provide progressive success and achievement on the part of the learner.

8. The involvement of disabled persons in community settings can best be achieved by a cooperative approach.

Potential resource persons who can exert a significant influence on the leisure life-style of a disabled person include: family members, education and recreation personnel, volunteers and staff of advocate associations, and municipal recreation and social service personnel.

Each of these individuals has an important role to play in developing the skills and abilities necessary for the disabled individual to maximize unobligated time. The approach to leisure skills development illustrated by this text requires and provides for meaningful involvement from *all* persons concerned with this process. While the assessment procedures and certain adaptation techniques lend themselves naturally to formal educational and recreative settings, family members, peers, and others could readily become involved in supplementing and reinforcing leisure skills instruction in home and community settings. In Chapter 10 numerous case studies provide ample suggestions for this process.

EMERGING ROLES OF LEISURE EDUCATION SPECIALISTS

Since this text reflects a novel and innovative approach to leisure education for the disabled person, application of the concepts presented will require a substantial shift in the roles and orientations of educational and recreational specialists. The following trends are illustrative of several of these new service functions and challenges.

1. Duties such as planning and providing mass diversional activities and coordinating special events will decrease in favor of the provision of individualized leisure and educational programming.

As the ability to function independently in the leisure sphere of life becomes one of the primary goals for persons returning from institutions, a dramatic shift will occur in the content of leisure services in residential facilities. Traditional duties associated with providing special events, spectator sports, and entertainment will cease to be the forté of residential leisure service personnel. Rather, institutional staff will perform assessment, evaluation, and instructional functions related to the provision of comprehensive leisure education curricula.

2. The medical model will be replaced by more appropriate orientations to leisure services for developmentally disabled persons.

According to Wolfensberger (1972), objectionable characteristics of the medical model as applied to human services include its fostering of feelings of helplessness, dependency, and passivity, the suggestion that different principles apply to normal and abnormal behavior, and the implication that responsibility for behavior be removed from the affected individual. Techniques such as those presented here are in direct opposition to these negative assumptions. The leisure skills model illustrated here ensures that the individual learner assume a very active role in each step of learning a recreational activity. The assumptions concerning learning are that disabled persons are not "sick" and can master age–appropriate skills by learning smaller, progressive units of behavior.

3. Behavior techniques can and will be reconciled with the principle of normalization.

According to some critics of behavior modification, the practice is contrary to the principle of normalization because of the tendency of behavioral interventions to control the actions of the learner. Interestingly, Wolfensberger (1972, p. 140–44) suggests that the manner in which behavioral strategies are used rather than the procedure itself determines the degree to which control is exerted. Furthermore, while applied behavioral techniques are "more specific and objective" than practices that occur in daily life, behavior modification is compatible with normalization. Recommendations made by Wolfensberger on the basis of current literature concerning the application of behavior modification are that program goals, rationale for procedures used, reward systems, and target behaviors be explained and discussed with the learner. These principles should be the basis for leisure skills development for the severely disabled.

4. Recreation and special education personnel must adopt the roles of advocate and community liaison in ensuring the rights of disabled persons to participate in community leisure opportunities.

While equipping a disabled person with the leisure skills necessary for mainstream involvement is the vital first step in the recreation-integration process, other factors frequently need to be addressed before this goal can become a reality. Bushell and Kelley (1974) identify several additional functions that specialists must be prepared to perform relative to this process including:

A. Educating able-bodied participants about the needs of the disabled
B. Holding small group conferences to allay the apprehension of parents
C. Coordinating volunteers in car pool efforts
D. Teaching disabled participants how to use public transportation
E. Assisting in the scheduling of activities in accessible facilities
F. Applying for grant funding to support training and program efforts
G. Publicizing available public recreational activities

Organized interventions that can be undertaken by action groups of concerned professionals include providing advisory assistance to governmental and public recreational agencies concerning the needs of the disabled, mounting of surveys and public awareness campaigns, conducting accessibility studies of leisure facilities, and assessing local recreational opportunities (Lyons & Reynolds, 1978). As the commitment to normalization increases, therapeutic recreators and special educators will assume a major responsibility in interpreting the leisure needs of disabled persons to community recreation personnel and in actively assisting in efforts to meet those needs.

5. The question of transfer of training must be addressed by teachers of leisure skills.

As behavioral programming replaces diversional activities for disabled persons, the question of generalization or transfer of learning must be seriously addressed by leisure service personnel. Specifically, the skills taught to handicapped learners must transcend specific activities, instructional sessions, and leisure settings if normalization is to be achieved. Hutchison (1975) suggests the following means to maximize the transfer benefits of skill development programs:

A. Programs should be made meaningful and relevant for participants by providing a variety of skill-specific and age-appropriate activities from which to choose.
B. Situations including tasks, group composition, and physical settings in special programs should resemble integrated environments.
C. An emphasis should be placed on developing a variety of generalizable competencies.
D. Play should be included with training in each session.
E. Developmental programming that emphasizes individualized teaching, the observation of strengths and weaknesses of the learner, and sequential teaching should be employed.

F. Self-confidence should be instilled in the learner through progressive successes in training.

This text incorporates each of these principles by including an abundance of curricular offerings, providing concrete suggestions for programming in community environments, stressing generalizable competencies such as free play skills, breaking tasks into behavior units that are enjoyable to the learner, and applying appropriate reinforcement techniques to ensure that the learner develops self-confidence.

REFERENCES

Braaten, J. The integration of moderately retarded children into regular residential camps—a demonstration program. *Leisurability*, 1977, *4*(3), 27–32.

Burdette, C., & Miller, M. Mainstreaming in a municipal recreation department utilizing a continuum method. *Therapeutic Recreation Journal*, 1979, *13*(4), 41–47.

Bushell, S., & Kelley, J. D. *Providing community recreation opportunities for the disabled.* Champaign, IL: University of Illinois at Champaign-Urbana Cooperative Extension Service, 1974.

Forness, S. R. A transition model for placement of handicapped children in regular and special classes. *Contemporary Educational Psychology*, 1977, *2*, 37–49.

Gunn, S. L., & Peterson, C. A. *Therapeutic recreation program design: principles and procedures.* Englewood Cliffs, NJ: Prentice-Hall, 1978.

Guralnick, M. J. The value of integrating handicapped and nonhandicapped preschool children. *American Journal of Orthopsychiatry*, 1976, *46*, 236–245.

Harasymiw, S. J., & Horne, M. D. Integration of handicapped children: its effect on teacher attitudes. *Education*, 1975, *96*(2), 158–168.

Hayes, G. A. Philosophical ramifications of mainstreaming in recreation. *Therapeutic Recreation Journal*, 1978, *12*(2), 5–9.

Hensley, D. L. Guidelines for integrating mentally retarded children and youth into regular day and residential camps. *Leisurability*, 1979, 6(4), 4–10.

Hutchison, M. L. Maximizing transfer benefits of special programs. *Leisurability*, 1975, *2*(4), 2–9.

Hutchison, P., & Lord, J. *Recreation integration: Issues and alternatives in leisure services and community involvement.* Ottawa, Ontario, Canada: Leisurability Publications, Inc., 1979.

Kugel, R. B., & Wolfensberger, W. The normalization principle and its human management implications. Extracted from *Changing patterns in residential services for the mentally retarded.* Washington, DC: President's Committee on Mental Retardation, 1969.

Lyons, R. F., & Reynolds, R. P. *How to improve community leisure opportunities for disabled people.* Halifax, Nova Scotia, Canada: The Recreation Council for the Disabled in Nova Scotia, 1978.

Matthews, P. R. Recreation and the normalization of the mentally retarded. *Therapeutic Recreation Journal*, 1977, *11*(3), 112–114.

Peterson, N. L., & Haralick, J. G. Integration of handicapped and nonhandicapped preschoolers: An analysis of play behavior and social interaction. *Education and Training of the Mentally Retarded*, 1977, *12*(1), 235-245.

Pomeroy, J. The handicapped are out of hiding: Implications for community recreation. *Therapeutic Recreation Journal*, 1974, *8*(3), 120-128.

Reynolds, R. P. The changing role of leisure services in residential facilities: Implications and challenges. *Leisurability*, 1978, *5*(3), 34-38.

Reynolds, R. P. What is normalization and how can you do it? *Parks and Recreation*, 1979, *14*, 33-34.

Stensrud, C. Sequential recreation integration streams. *Leisurability*, 1978, *5*(2), 28-33.

Szymanski, D. J. PL 94-142: The education for all handicapped children act. *Therapeutic Recreation Journal*, 1976, *10*(1), 6-10.

Turnball, A. P., & Schulz, J. B. *Mainstreaming handicapped students: A guide for the classroom teacher*. Boston, MA: Allyn and Bacon, 1979.

Wehman, P., & Schleien, S. Assessment and selection of leisure skills for severely handicapped individuals. *Education and Training of the Mentally Retarded*, 1980, *15*(1), 50-56.

Witt, P. A. *Community leisure services and disabled individuals*. Washington, DC: Hawkins and Associates, 1977.

Wolfensberger, W. *The principle of normalization in human services*. Toronto, Canada: National Institute on Mental Retardation, 1972.

Chapter 2
LEISURE SKILLS ASSESSMENT

The assessment of leisure skills competencies is the initial step in beginning a recreation program that is appropriate for handicapped individuals. Assessment is a process that allows for identification and verification of the individual's entry level skills for participating in leisure education programs. Accurate assessment is important because it provides the benchmark for establishing the client's initial competencies and what his or her potential may be in different activity areas.

Leisure skills assessment must be viewed not only as a process that precedes instruction, but, instead, as an ongoing process that regularly provides feedback to the therapist or teacher. This feedback is necessary for communicating the effectiveness of the instructional techniques or the special activities employed. Assessment also provides important information for administrators, parents, and others not directly involved in service delivery as to the impact of the program on clients.

An optimal approach to leisure skills assessment does not rely solely on one measure. Multiple sources of data, such as parental perceptions of client satisfaction, increase in repertoire of activities, and improvement in the other skill areas, enchance the status of the leisure program. It is advisable to assess other curriculum areas (i.e., motor, social, communication) for positive changes as well as improvements in specific leisure skills areas. Usually, concurrent changes will be observed.

In this chapter several forms of assessment are discussed. Since many leisure assessment tools involve paper and pencil measures and client preference-evaluations, a brief description of the leading tools in this area is presented first. Following this information, which is directed toward mildly handicapped individuals, is a discussion of several behavioral variables that should be assessed in recreation settings. This type of assessment calls for direct observation and recording of specific leisure activities; it is also characterized by ongoing assessment in a variety of environments, such as home, classroom, and community facilities. From these discussions of assessment, a model of selection of leisure skills is outlined. The assessment data collected are a precursor to leisure skills selection.

EVALUATING LEISURE SKILLS ASSESSMENT GUIDES

In evaluating different leisure skills assessment tools, it is necessary to consider several criteria. They are:

Table 1. Leisure skill assessment tools

Leisure assessment instruments	1 Response mode	2 Target population	3 Norm ref.	3 Criterion ref.	4 Reliability	5 Ease of administration	6 Validity	7 Individual vs. group
1. Avocational Activities Inventory	S	EMR		X	Good	QA	Good	I
2. Bogan's Group Assessment	D	All		X		TC		I/G
3. Comprehensive Evaluation in Recreational Therapy Scale (CERT)	D	Short-term psychiatric		X	Good	TC		I
4. Constructive Leisure Activity Survey (CLAS)	E	Normal		X		QA		I
5. I Can	D	TMR—children		X	Good	QA	Good	I/G
6. Davis' Recreational Directors' Observational Report	D	Psychiatric		X		TC,		I
7. Iowa Leisure Education Program	D, S	Hospitalized		X		TC		I
8. Joswiak's Leisure Counseling Assessment Form	E, S	Developmentally disabled		X		TC	Good	I
9. Knox, Hurff, & Takata Deaf-Blind Assessment	S	Deaf-blind birth–adolescence		X		QA		I
10. Leisure Activities Blank (LAB)	E	Normal	X		Good	QA	Good	I

11.	Leisure Interest Inventory (LII)	E	Normal	X		Good
12.	Linear Model for Individual Treatment in Recreation (LMIT)	E, D	Developmentally disabled		X	Good	TC
13.	Leisure Skills Curriculum Assessment Inventory (LSCDD)	D, S	Developmentally disabled		X		TC
14.	Minimum Objective System (MOS)	D, S	Severly handicapped		X	Good	QA
15.	Mirenda Leisure Interest Finder	E	Normal intelligence	X			QA
16.	Recreation Therapy Assessment	D	Nonambulatory, adult		X		TC
17.	Self-Leisure Interest Profile (SLIP)	E	Normal intelligence		X		QA
18.	Sonoma County Organization for the Retarded Assessment System (SCOR)	E, S	Developmentally disabled		X	Good	TC
19.	State of Ohio Curriculum Guide for Moderately Mentally Retarded Learners	D, S	TMR		X		TC
20.	Toward Competency: A Guide for Individualized Instruction	E, S	All special populations		X		TC
21.	Vineland Social Maturity Scale	S	All	X		Good	QA

Column headers all yield I.

Key: 1, Response mode: E, examinee; D, direct observation by examiner; S, staff/parent. 5, Ease of administration: QA, quickly administered; TC, time-consuming. 7, Individual versus group assessment: I, individual; G, group.

17

1. Norm-referenced versus criterion-referenced tools
2. What population the tool was designed for
3. Ease and practicality of repeated administrations
4. Type of response mode (i.e., client versus direct observation versus staff/parent)
5. Validity of instrument

Listed below are several leisure guides. They are discussed in the context of how they relate to the above criteria.

Several instruments have been developed to assist the practitioner in assessing the functioning levels and leisure skills repertoires of the client. Such tools act as guides for selecting the overall goals of therapy for each individual, and at times, for groups. The assessment instruments described below frequently vary in the populations for which they were developed and in the specificity of the behaviors evaluated.

Some of the most widely used tools concern themselves with the individual's overall behavioral functioning. The Vineland Social Maturity Scale deals with a wide variety of populations. Items are categorized by developmental level and vary from simple motor tasks such as grasping an object, to more advanced social skills such as making telephone calls.

Other assessment inventories may be more specific as to the skills evaluated and the populations targeted. The Leisure Activities Blank (LAB) lists 120 activities and the extent of past participation and intended future involvement in those activities. The LAB, which is now available in standardized published form, does not have established norms for various exceptional groups such as the physically handicapped.

The Linear Model for Individual Treatment in Recreation (LMIT) is a popular and detailed programmatic model that, like the Vineland Social Maturity Scale, measures overall behavioral competency. Developed for the developmentally disabled persons, LMIT assesses specific competencies in six developmental areas and consequently determines the client's priority needs.

Oftentimes, assessment tools are developed as part of a curriculum package to facilitate appropriate skill selection. For example, the Sonoma County Organization for the Retarded Assessment System (SCOR) was recently developed as an auxiliary assessment instrument for the SCOR Curriculum. It exists to initiate programs for developmentally disabled persons that promote independence, productivity, self-respect, and deinstitutionalization. To meet these goals, the SCOR assessment identifies program areas, monitors client progress, as well as assesses independent living skills. The I Can Curriculum, Minimum Objective System, and Leisure Skills Curriculum for Developmentally Disabled Persons also provide assessment tools that aid the programmer in individualized and appropriate skill selection.

Some tools are administered by having the client or examinee respond to the items (e.g., Mirenda Leisure Interest Finder), as opposed to the frequently utilized direct observation technique (e.g., State of Ohio Curriculum Guide for Moderately Mentally Retarded Learners). But many times, the intellectual functioning level of the client does not allow for direct examinee response. In these cases, the examiner may have to collect data from those who are in daily contact with the client such as parents and staff. The Iowa Leisure Education Program Assessment Form uses staff members working with the clients and family as sources of information for assessment purposes.

Sometimes it is desirable and/or necessary to assess a person's leisure needs and interests as a group member. This is because the recreational therapist must program for large numbers of participants simultaneously, making it literally impossible to assess on an individual basis. In addition, the composition of a leisure-related activity may entail a group effort or response, and therefore may require an assessment instrument that examines the group's functioning as a whole. Bogan's Group Assessment makes selected observations and assumptions concerning the group. These data are joined together to explain the nature of the participants and relate to the action that could and should be taken. The I Can Curriculum offers a "Class Performance Score Sheet" that allows the practitioner to easily and objectively assess each individual's ability and entry status on the targeted activity. This group assessment is the basis for planning individualized instructional activities for the daily lesson plan. See Table 1 for a list of 19 leisure assessment instruments and their criteria characteristics.

BEHAVIORAL VARIABLES FOR LEISURE ASSESSMENT

When initiating a leisure skills program for more severely impaired participants, a direct behavioral approach is necessary. Initial assessment will help determine which skills the participant can perform independently and which skills require verbal, gestural, or physical assistance. Unfortunately, most of the previously reviewed leisure skills inventories are not sensitive to the unique needs and problems of severely and profoundly handicapped persons. Although work is underway in this area (e.g., Wehman & Schleien, 1979), at this point it is necessary to use leisure skills inventories designed for higher-functioning individuals or recreation activity guides with activities or skills that have not been task analyzed. The variables below provide numerous areas for assessment.

Proficiency of Leisure Skills: Task Analytic Assessment

An initial consideration in beginning a recreation program is: *Does the individual know how to interact with the materials?* Stated another way, when given leisure skills materials, can the participant use them appropriately? If not, then systematic instruction is required.

What is required for evaluating leisure skills proficiency is task analytic assessment (Knapczyk, 1975). An instructional objective must be written for a given material. The objective should reflect the specific skill that the teacher or therapist wants the individual to learn. An example of a task analytic assessment for tossing a frisbee is provided in Table 2. This table contains an instructional objective, a task analysis for tossing a frisbee, and the verbal cue provided during the assessment. The recording form indicates that the first five days of assessment (baseline) Robert performed a total of three, three, two, four, and four steps independently. This indicates that instruction should begin at step four in the task analysis.

There are multiple advantages to this type of observational assessment. First, the information collected about the individual on this particular leisure skill helps the teacher to pinpoint the exact point where instruction should begin. In this way, the participant does not receive instruction on skills in which he is already proficient. Second, this facilitates step-by-step individualized instruction for persons with complex learning problems. Evaluation of the individual's proficiency with different objects/materials over an extended period of time will also be more objective and precise, and will be less subject to teacher bias.

Duration of Activity

If the individual has some degree of proficiency with leisure materials as Reid, Willis, Jarman, & Brown (1978) found, then the instructional var-

Table 2. Task analytic assessment for tossing a frisbee

Step	M	T	W	Th	F
1. Extend hand downward toward frisbee.	+	+	+	+	+
2. Curl fingers underneath frisbee.	+	+	+	+	+
3. Position thumb on top edge of frisbee.	+	+	−	+	+
4. Apply inward pressure with fingers and thumb to grasp frisbee firmly.	−	−	−	+	+
5. Bend at elbow, raising frisbee to chest.	−	−	−	−	−
6. Hold frisbee parallel to ground.	−	−	−	−	−
7. Bring frisbee inward toward nondominant side of body.	−	−	−	−	−
8. Quickly extend elbow outward away from body.	−	−	−	−	−
9. Snap wrist outward and extend fingers to release frisbee.	−	−	−	−	−
10. Toss frisbee 2 feet.	−	−	−	−	−
11. Toss frisbee 3 feet.	−	−	−	−	−
12. Toss frisbee 4 feet.	−	−	−	−	−
13. Toss frisbee 5 feet.	−	−	−	−	−

Table 3. Initial object assessment

Leisure skill object	Minutes/seconds engaged with object	Type of object
1. Waterpaints		
2. Record player		
3. Plants		
4. Goldfish		
5. Ball		
6. Magazine		
7. Box of Crackerjacks		
8. Frisbee		
9. Viewfinder		
10. Pinball machine		

iable of interest may be the duration or length of time the participant engages in activity. This is assessed by recording the amount of time the individual engages in different activities.

Since this may be an extremely time-consuming measure to use with several individuals at once, the teacher may elect to observe only half the participants one day and the other half the next. Another option is to record activity involvement only twice a week instead of daily.

The length of time spent in independent leisure activity is particularly important to assess because of its relevance to most home situations where parents cannot constantly occupy time with their handicapped child. A frequently heard request from many parents is to teach the child to play independently, thereby relieving the family of continual supervision. A careful assessment of the child's duration of leisure activity before instruction will help the teacher and parents set realistic independent leisure goals for the child. Table 3 presents a sample data collection sheet.

Discriminating Between Appropriate Versus Inappropriate Object Manipulation

Another assessment issue faced by teachers and researchers is differentiation between appropriate actions with objects versus actions that would not be considered appropriate. Several play studies have failed to address this issue (Burney, Russell, & Shores, 1977; Favell & Cannon, 1977; Wehman, 1977). Inappropriate play actions have typically been considered those behaviors that are harmful or destructive to the child, peers, or materials. However, many profoundly retarded and autistic children will exhibit high rates of repetitive self-stimulatory behavior with toys, (i.e., banging, pounding, slamming), that are not necessarily harmful or destructive, yet still inappropriate. Furthermore, the problem is compounded since banging or slamming actions with certain objects may be appropriate. Many children will do unusual things with toys that *might* be considered appropriate by other observers (Goetz & Baer, 1973).

Consequently, teachers are faced with how to assess the qualitative nature of object manipulation. There are several ways of coping with this difficulty. The first one involves using two to three observers periodically and having these observers rate the appropriateness of the action. Objective judging provides a system of checks and balances for the teacher.

A second method of assessing appropriateness of object manipulation is to identify the principle actions that a nonhandicapped child of comparable mental age might do with each object (Fredericks, Baldwin, Grove, Moore, Riggs, & Lyons, 1978). These actions may serve as guidelines.

Identifying a number of fine motor categories for object manipulation is yet another means of coding the qualitative nature of responses. This requires generating a fine motor classification system that observers can use as a basis for recording actions. Tilton and Ottinger (1964) provide nine categories that are self-explanatory, and that are identified after extensive observational analysis of normal, trainable retarded, and autistic children. These are listed below:

1. Repetitive manual manipulation
2. Oral contacts
3. Pounding
4. Throwing
5. Pushing or pulling
6. Personalized toy use
7. Manipulation of movable parts
8. Separation of parts of toys
9. Combinational use of toys

Schleien, Kiernan, and Wehman (1980) operationally defined what they considered to be high and low quality behavior and inappropriate social behavior during leisure skills programming at a group home. They successfully increased the percentage of high quality leisure behavior among six participants at the residential community agency by implementing a program consisting of leisure counseling, skill training, and exposure to new materials. The leisure quality definitions used for the program follow:

High Quality Leisure Behavior (HQ)
    Goal-directed recreational activity (includes goal-directed conversation relevant to leisure)
    Chronologically age-appropriate

Appropriate use of materials and/or equipment in a manner consistent with correct level of training
(*Note:* All criteria listed above must be met in order for behavior to be considered high quality.)

Low Quality Leisure Behavior (LQ)
Use of leisure-related materials and/or equipment in a manner inconsistent with present level of training
Sitting or lying passively without participating in an activity
Watching television
Smoking without additional activity
Solitary engagement in appropriate activity that necessarily requires more than one participant

Inappropriate Social Behavior (I)
Inappropriate use of materials
Use of chronologically age-inappropriate materials (determined by manufacturer's recommended age level)
Violently aggressive verbal or physical behavior
Non-goal-directed, nonfunctional, purposeless behavior (e.g., wandering aimlessly around home, spinning in circles)
Purposeless, nonsensical conversation (e.g., speaking to oneself, speaking to another individual in a socially unacceptable manner, echolalic or perseverative speech)
Stereotypic behavior (e.g., body rocking, self-stimulation)
Behavior out of context

A momentary time sampling assessment technique employed in order to record quality of leisure behavior appears in Table 4.

Leisure Preference Evaluation

Assessing favorite leisure activities is an important step in initiating a recreation program. The goal in this process is to identify which, if any, activities are preferred by the participant. This is a fairly easy task. By employing duration assessment, the amount of minutes/seconds spent with each leisure material can be recorded. This observation and recording should take place for at least a week.

A second means of assessing leisure preference is through presenting a small number of different materials and determining the amount of time before the participant responds. This is referred to as a *latency* measure of behavior.

McCall (1974) has used latency as a measure of the length of time that elapsed before infants acted on a variety of objects that were presented. Each of the objects possessed different stimulus attributes such as configural complexity or sound potential. Through measuring passage

Table 4. Leisure skill observational recording sheet

Instructions: Observe three participants at times specified on reinforcement schedule and then record quality of participants' behavior at that moment. If participant is exhibiting high quality leisure behavior (HQ), socially reinforce and participate with each for 30 seconds. If three participants are exhibiting HQ, socially reinforce and participate with each for 20 seconds. Immediately following minute of reinforcement, record quality of behavior (HQ, LQ, I) for each participant in appropriate box. *Only* reinforce HQ leisure behavior. During 10-minute nonreinforced probes, record quality of first participant's behavior at that moment. Then 15 seconds later, record quality of second participant's behavior. Continue recording cycle (one participant at a time) for 10 minutes.

Specialist's name _____ Date _____ Day of week _____

Participant's name	1	2	3	4	5	6	7	8	9	10	11	12	13	14	15	16	17
1																	
2																	
3																	

	18	19	20	21	22	23	24	25	26	27	28	29	30	31	32	33	34
1																	
2																	
3																	

	35	36	37	38	39	40	41	42	43	44	45	46	47	48	49	50	51
1																	
2																	
3																	

Participant's leisure behaviors	
1	
2	
3	

of time until a response, teachers may be able to evaluate the relative attractiveness of and preferences for certain materials with severely handicapped individuals.

Frequency of Interactions

For many severely handicapped children, an important instructional goal is to initiate and sustain interactions with peers more frequently. Several delayed children each playing in isolation during free play is a relatively common occurence. (Fredericks, Baldwin, Grove, Moore, Riggs, & Lyons, 1978). When this happens, the potential benefits of social interaction are not accrued.

One way of assessing social interaction is a simple count of the number of times one child 1) initiates an interaction, 2) receives an interaction, and 3) terminates interaction. Duration assessment may be used to measure the length of the interaction between peers and also between the child and adults in the room.

A second means of gathering more information on social interactions is the coding of specific types of interactions. Carney and her associates (1977) have detailed the following social interaction skills:

- A. Receives interaction
    1. Receives hug
    2. Returns smile
    3. Gives object to other who has requested it
    4. Returns a greeting
    5. "Receives" cooperative play
    6. Answers questions
    7. Recognizes peers, teachers by name
    8. Shows approval
    9. Discriminates appropriate time, place, situation
- B. Initiates interaction
    1. Greets another person
    2. Requests objects from another person
    3. Initiates cooperative play
    4. Seeks approval
    5. Seeks affiliation with familiar person
    6. Helps one who has difficulty manipulating environment
    7. Initiates conversation
- C. Sustains interactions
    1. Attends to ongoing cooperative activity
    2. Sustains conversation
- D. Terminates interactions
    1. Terminates cooperative play activity
    2. Terminates conversation

This sequence provides an important step toward detailing the specific skills that teachers should be attempting to elicit in delayed children. In addition to providing sequence, these skills may be task analyzed and the child's proficiency on selected behaviors assessed. These four categories of interaction can be employed to code the qualitative nature of the interaction (Hamre-Nietupski & Williams, 1977).

Direction of Interaction

Analyzing to whom interactions are directed may also be helpful in assessing which individuals in the play environment are reinforcing to the child. As Beveridge and his colleagues (1978) observed, child-teacher interactions occur more frequently than child-child interactions, especially with severely delayed children. Structured intervention by an adult is usually required to increase child-child interactions (Shores, Hester, & Strain, 1976).

When making home visits and observing the child playing at home with siblings or with neighborhood children, the direction of interactions should be assessed. This should be done not only with handicapped children, but also with nonhandicapped peers. This type of behavioral analysis can be revealing since most nonhandicapped children do not include handicapped children in play unless prompted and reinforced by adults (e.g., Apolloni & Cooke, 1978).

Free Play Assessment

In some cases, there may be little interest or time to collect the specific types of information that have been discussed. Some teachers may want to consider using a simpler method of assessing the level of free play at which the child is functioning (Wehman & Marchant, 1978).

With this strategy, the teacher clearly defines the types of behaviors that are characteristic of the different developmental levels of play. For example, in the autistic play stage, characteristic behaviors might include not touching or physically acting on any play materials during free play periods or nonfunctional repetitive actions for long periods of time. Independent play might be considered as any appropriate play behaviors that were exhibited alone or away from other peers. Cooperative or social play would be another skill level in the basic developmental sequence and would include such skills as physical or verbal interaction with other peers and teachers (Fredericks et al., 1978).

This assessment strategy is convenient and economical in terms of time expended; it allows for easy collection of fairly accurate information provided the categories are clearly defined and, therefore, easy to discriminate. This type of behavioral assessment does not, however, capture many of the collateral skills that are clearly associated with play skills development such as fine motor skills, changes in emotionality, and social behavior.

A MODEL FOR SELECTION OF LEISURE SKILLS

While the leisure skills variables discussed above are important in the program development process, it is equally important to systematically review criteria for skill selection. The nature of the assessment data and factors involved constitute the initial skill selection. These criteria must be carefully assessed before beginning a program. They include the participant's leisure skills preference, functioning level and physical characteristics, the age appropriateness of the skills, participant's access to materials, and the quality and support available in the home environment. A sequence of questions that the teacher should ask in reviewing skills for instruction is listed below. These guidelines are helpful in determining the range of skills that may be selected.

Preference	What skills does the client already demonstrate?
Functioning	What are the client's capabilities and educational needs?
Physical characteristics	What physical characteristics does the client have or lack that may interfere with leisure skills development?
Age-appropriateness	Are the skills that have been selected for instruction the type of skills that nonhandicapped peers might engage in?
Access to materials	What is the client's access to materials (financial resources, transportation, etc.)?
Support of home environment	What persons are available in the home or neighborhood environment to reinforce leisure skills development?

Leisure Skills Preference

The initial question to consider in determining which leisure skills to select for instruction is: *How does the individual presently spend his free time?* Stated another way, what leisure skills does the individual currently engage in?

There are several reasons for using this as an indicator. One, it may provide the teacher with insights into the type or category of leisure activities (e.g., games, sports, hobbies, toys) that the participant enjoys. Second, the activity may be used as a reinforcer for other new leisure skills that are the objectives of instruction. Third, and perhaps most important, it allows the teacher to determine what the participant can already do and at what level of proficiency. Through placement of a variety of leisure skills materials (Reid et al., 1978) and task analytic assessment (Knapczyk, 1975; Wehman, 1979), a determination can be made of object preferences, and quality of performance with different materials.

As an illustration, consider the placement of a variety of hobby-type materials (i.e., goldfish, record player, waterpaints). The teacher can observe and record which materials were preferred by assessing those that were selected, how proficient the individual was with the material, and for what period of time he engaged in its use. Similar assessments might be made with toys, gross motor recreational equipment, such as playground equipment, and simple card or board games. This can also be done with several materials from each leisure category. The data collection sheet presented earlier in Table 3 represents a means of assessing durations.

Although this type of assessment may be helpful in determining the participant's leisure skills preference, this does not tell the teacher *what* materials and/or activities to make available. With the large number of leisure skills that might be engaged in, this becomes a critical question.

Functioning Level and Specific Educational Needs

The participant's present functioning level will greatly affect the choice of materials and activities that should be provided for assessment. Consideration of the individual's abilities across major curriculum areas cannot be ignored. The factors in Table 5 must be evaluated in determining which leisure skills to target for instruction.

Although the questions asked in Table 5 are certainly not comprehensive, they do reflect the points that must be considered in determining which materials and activities are appropriate for assessment. Behavioral checklists and guides such as the Learning Accomplishment Profile or the Minimum Objective System (Williams & Fox, 1977), provide considerably more detail. This is necessary for determining the approximate level at which the individual is functioning.

The questions answered by this type of screening assessment are:

A. What behaviors is this individual currently capable of? and
B. What are the behaviors or component skills that make up the leisure activities that are targeted for instruction?

A general parity or agreement between these two questions must be made so that the leisure skill selection will not be too easy or too hard for the individual.

Consider the following illustration of this process. Susan's IEP indicates that at her present performance level she is unable to attend for a period longer than three seconds, yet demonstrates competent fine motor behavior (e.g., able to grasp and pick up objects, push and pull objects, squeeze, release, and transfer). She is usually withdrawn and stays in the corner engaging in high rates of self-stimulation, (i.e. twisting string or picking up scraps of paper from floor and putting them in her mouth). Susan's teacher has provided a variety of card and board games for Susan and the other students in the play area. However, Susan does not play appropriately with the games. Her approximate functioning level is not at parity with the skills required in the board games. This is one example of how capricious skill selection can interfere with the individual's leisure skills development.

Table 5. Client functioning level representative skills for consideration

I. Expressive and Receptive Language
How long does the participant attend to a task?
Is participant able to focus attention on a simple task if other stimuli are at a minumum?
Does the participant express self verbally, gesturally, or not at all?
How does the participant interact with authority figures?
Does the participant have difficulty determining which are important aspects of the task?
Does the participant understand one-step versus two-step instructions?

II. Physical/Motor Characteristics
Does the participant hold his head up?
Does the participant sit on the floor unsupported?
Does the participant turn his head to watch a moving object?
Does the participant have a functional pincer versus palmar grasp?
Does the participant have full use of at least one arm?
Does the participant reach for an object when placed in front of the body? When placed under barrier and out of sight?
Does the participant ambulate independently?
Does the participant use a prosthetic device in his daily living?

III. Social Skills
What is participant's level of play interaction with others (solitary, parallel, cooperative, competitive)?
Does the participant exhibit positive affect during leisure activity?
Does the participant display the ability to take turns and share materials?
What is the nature of participant's physical contact with others (appropriate versus abusive)?
Does the participant draw attention away from activity by inappropriate actions or complete withdrawal?
What is the participant's attitude toward winning and losing?

If the IEP committee has done a good job of initial assessment and instructional objectives have been clearly specified, then selection of leisure skills may be facilitated through interrelating IEP objectives with leisure skills goals.

Physical Characteristics

In most cases, new behavior can be developed and maintained in individuals who are functioning at low developmental levels. This is done through behavioral training techniques (e.g., Kazdin, 1975). However, the participant's physical characteristics will directly affect selection of leisure skills for instruction. Individuals with severe motor impairments, such as an inability to hold the head up, extreme spasticity, or uncontrollable seizures, present additional problems in the identification of appropriate leisure skills for instruction.

What is important to remember with this factor is that even though such physical disabilities are rarely reversible, they need not interfere with leisure skills programming (Williams, Briggs, & Williams, 1979). For example, the child with spasticity in arms and hands might enter into a game of moving a ping pong ball back and forth through use of a head pointer. This same skill might also facilitate scanning and head pointer control on a communication board. The spastic child who is unable to use standard size materials could initially use oversize pieces in a table game (Wehman & Schleien, 1979). The adaptations are endless and require only a teacher's creativity and an occupational/physical therapist's knowledge of motor development (Williams et al., 1979).

Age-Appropriate Level of Skill

Another variable that must be considered in the assessment and skill selection process is how age-appropriate the skill is. The principal question to consider is: *Would a nonhandicapped individual of comparable chronological age engage in this activity in his or her free time?* Severely handicapped adults on the floor pushing a toy truck around or playing with a dollhouse are examples of inappropriate skill selection.

This is, admittedly, a difficult area, especially with adolescents and adults. Very little leisure skills research has been reported with this age population. The answer to this problem is usually found in a detailed breakdown of the skill into very small behaviors. For example, the prospect of teaching plant care to a severely or profoundly handicapped individual may appear remote. However, if this hobby is divided into several skills (e.g. putting soil in pot, putting flower in soil, putting holder on plant, watering plant), and each skill is task-analyzed, then learning problems will be reduced (Wehman & Schleien, 1978). This is especially true for those teachers who understand how to implement shaping and chaining instructional procedures (Kazdin, 1975).

Because of the difficulty in identifying age-appropriate skills, Table 6 has been provided. This table presents representative skills in categories of object manipulation, hobbies, sports, and games for adolescents and adults that may be appropriate for instruction.

Access to Materials and Events

The most capable individual will have difficulty engaging in a variety of leisure activities without access to materials or events. At the least, this involves transportation and some financial resources. This poses the question: *Can the participant get to community events, and if unemployed, does he or she have the money to make necessary purchases?* Although leisure activities can be engaged in without money (i.e., building a snowman) usually some funds are necessary for new materials and replenishing old materials.

There are other factors to consider as well. For example, initiating a social encounter may be difficult without knowledge of how to use a telephone (Nietupski & Williams, 1974) or if no phone is available. Interaction with toys or other play objects at home is impossible without funds to purchase new ones when old ones are destroyed. Similarly, many residents in state facilities have difficulty operating the television or stereo that is placed 8 to 10 feet above the floor.

In short, a careful assessment of what to teach must include a look at the amount and type of materials available, the proximity and physical design of local recreational facilities, the ease of transportation, and the availability of skilled recreational personnel to provide the training. An analysis of these variables will, at a minimum, facilitate a decision concerning how broad a program to establish. It will also help identify what areas need more adaptation and planning. Table 7 provides a summary of the variables that must be considered.

Home Environment

Perhaps the most critical factor in leisure skill selection is evaluation of the home and neighborhood environment. The age of the individual's

Table 6. Representative objects, games, hobbies, and sports appropriate for severely handicapped adolescent and adult leisure skills instruction

I. Object Manipulation
Representative objects:
Camera, Dice, Flashlight, Frisbee, Guitar, Handgrippers, Hammer, Medicine ball, Scissors, Telephone, Vending machine.

II. Games
Representative games:
a. Board and table games—Bingo, Checkers, Crossword puzzles, Darts, Football, Ping Pong, Pinball, Pool, Scrabble, Tic-Tac-Toe.
b. Motor games Arm Wrestle, Charades, Finger (Thumb) Wrestling, Jump Rope, Tetherball, Tug of War.
c. Musical Rhythmic games—Hokey Pokey, Limbo, Name That Tune.
d. Card games—Concentration, I Doubt It, Old Maid, Slap Jack, War.

III Hobbies
Representative hobbies:
Camping, Cooking, Decorating for social events, Leatherwork, Pet care, Plant care, Spectator Leisure, Community events, String art, Sunbathing, Woodwork.

IV. Sports
Representative sports:
Badminton, Bowling, Fishing, Horseshoes, Shuffleboard, Jogging, Weight training, Winter sports.

parents, the presence of siblings or other relatives in the home, the type of home, and the attitude of other home members will greatly influence the variety and independence of leisure activities engaged in.

Location of the home also affect the selection process. Urban living presents different problems than living in sparsely populated rural areas. Sensitivity of local communities and neighborhood members to handicapped persons will also be reflected in the amount of funds that are appropriated for therapeutic recreation programming. Table 8 is a checklist of factors to consider in evaluating the home environment for leisure skill selection.

The willingness of parents and other family members to follow through school training programs is important as well. Marchant and Wehman (1979) found that demonstration and behavior rehearsal with a foster mother of a severely retarded child was instrumental in generalizing

Table 7. Participants' access to materials and resources

I. Amount and Type of Materials Available
   A. What toys, games, or other recreational materials/equipment are available to the participant in home, school, or work environments?
   B. Can recreation materials/equipment be borrowed by community agencies (e.g., public library, university curriculum center)?
   C. Are funds available in the home, school, or work environments to purchase additional recreation equipment?
   D. Does the participant have access to a record player, radio, or other equipment for musical enjoyment?

II. Proximity and Physical Design of Community Recreation Opportunities and Ease of Transportation
   A. Are leisure service agencies offering recreation opportunities to special populations?
   B. Is the participant making use of the recreation services that are readily available in the community?
   C. Can the participant utilize nonadapted playground equipment?
   D. How close are the local park and playground to the participant's home?
   E. Is activity for the participant in the community recreation program significantly hampered because of architectural or attitudinal barriers, or lack of appropriate programming?
   F. Is adequate transportation available for the participant to get to community recreation facilities?

III. Availability of Skilled Recreational Personnel
   A. Are the community recreation personnel working within the community able to facilitate participation of persons with special needs?
   B. Is there a trained recreation consultant/staff available to help develop leisure programs for special populations?

Table 8. Client home environment

> The participant lives with _____.
> Relationships and ages of other persons in home _____
>
> How does the participant utilize has free time at home?
> Does the participant utilize his leisure time independently or with assistance in the home?
> What leisure activities and interests are enjoyed by others in home?
> How many hours per day do housemates/siblings spend with participant?
> Do housemates have any natural (e.g., athletics, musical ability) or learned (e.g., cooking, tools) talents?
> How is the participant perceived by himself and by family members?
> What are the present attitudes toward recreation and leisure held by the participant's family members?
> Does the participant reside in an urban or rural area?
> What is the general attitude of the neighborhood toward integration of handicapped persons into community programs?
> Does the pariticipant interact with others in the neighborhood?

table game skills from the classroom to the home. This shows that parent-professional partnership is vital to maintenance of a leisure activity repertoire in severely handicapped individuals.

SUMMARY

The purpose of this chapter has been to describe several types of leisure skills competency areas that can be assessed in severely handicapped individuals. These include the proficiency with which objects or materials were engaged, the length of self-initiated action, materials preference by clients, and frequency and direction of social interactions.

In the second half of the chapter guidelines for selecting leisure skills were presented. A variety of areas were identified as critical to the skill selection process. Client preference for different materials, functioning level, age-appropriateness of activity, and support of the home environment were among the principle criteria clusters.

When these assessment and skill guidelines are provided in conjunction with logically sequenced recreation curriculum and instructional technology, the application of the systematic instruction process to leisure skills development is complete. What remains is the continued development, field testing, and validation of leisure skills curricula. The items sequenced in these curricula will then serve as appropriate criterion-referenced skills for assessment.

REFERENCES

Apolloni, T., & Cooke, T. Integrated programming at the infant, toddler, and preschool levels. In: M. Guralnick (Ed.), *Early intervention and the integration of handicapped and nonhandicapped children*. Baltimore: University Park Press, 1978.

Berkson, G., & Davenport, R. K. Stereotyped movements of mental defectives. I. Initial Survey. *American Journal of Mental Deficiency*, 1962, *66*, 849–852.

Beveridge, M., Spencer, J., & Miller, P. Language and social behavior in severely educationally subnormal children. *British Journal of Social and Clinical Psychology*, 1978, *17*(1), 75–83.

Burney, J., Russell, B., & Shores, R. Developing social responses in two profoundly retarded children. *AAESPH Review*, 1977, *2*(2), 53–63.

Carney, I., Clobuciar, A., Corley, E., Wilcox, B., Bigler, J., Fleisler, L., Pany, D., & Turner, P. Social interaction in severely handicapped students. In: *The Severely and Profoundly Handicapped Child*. Springfield, IL: State Department of Education, 1977.

Favell, J. Reduction of stereotypes by reinforcement of toy play. *Mental Retardation*, 1973, *11*(4), 24–27.

Favell, J., & Cannon, P. R. Evaluation of entertainment materials for severely retarded persons. *American Journal of Mental Deficiency*, 1977, *81*(4), 357–361.

Fredericks, H. D., Baldwin, V., Grove, D., Moore, W., Riggs, C., & Lyons, B. Integrating the moderately and severely handicapped preschool child into a normal day care setting. In: M. Guralnick (Ed.), *Early intervention and the integration of handicapped and nonhandicapped children*. Baltimore: University Park Press, 1978.

Gable, R., Hendrickson, J., & Strain, P. S. Assessment modification, and generalization of social interaction among severely retarded multihandicapped children. *Education and Training of the Mentally Retarded*, 1978, *13*(3), 279–286.

Goetz, E., & Baer, D. Social control of form diversity and the emergence of new forms in children's blockbuilding. *Journal of Applied Behavior Analysis*, 1973, *6*, 209–217.

Hamre-Nietupski, S., & Williams, W. W. Implementation of selected sex education and social skills programs with severely handicapped students. *Education and Training of the Mentally Retarded*, 1977, *12*(4), 364–372.

Kazdin, A. E. *Behavior modification in applied settings*. Homewood, IL: Dorsey Press, 1975.

Knapczyk, D. Task analytic assessment of severe learning problems. *Education and Training of the Mentally Retarded*, 1975, *16*, 24–27.

Marchant, J., & Wehman, P. Teaching table games to severely retarded children. *Mental Retardation*, 1979, *17*, 150–152.

McCall, R. Exploratory manipulation and play in the human infant. *Monographs of the Society for Research on Child Development*. Chicago, IL: University of Chicago Press, 1974.

Morris, R., & Dolker, M. Developing cooperative play in socially withdrawn retarded children. *Mental Retardation*, 1974, *12*(6), 24–27.

Nietupski, J., & Williams, W. W. Teaching severely handicapped students to use the telephone to initiate selected recreational activities and to respond appropriately to telephone requests to engage in selected recreational activities. In: L. Brown, W. Williams, & T. Crowner (Eds.), *A Collection of Papers and Programs Related to Public School Services for Severely Handicapped Students*. Madison, WI: Madison Public Schools, 1977.

Quilitch, H. R., & Delongchamp, G. D. Increasing recreational participation of institutional neuro-psychiatric residents. *Therapeutic Recreation*, 1974, *8*, 56–57.

Quilitch, H. R., & Risley, T. The effects of play materials on social play. *Journal of Applied Behavior Analysis*, 1973, *6*, 573–578.

Reid, D., Willis, B., Jarman, P., & Brown, K. Increasing leisure activity of physically disabled retarded persons through modifying resource availability. *AAESPH Review*, 1978, *3*(2), 78–93.

Schleien, S., Kiernan, J., & Wehman, P. Education and training of training of the mentally retarded. In press.

Shores, R., Hester, P., & Strain, P. S. The effects of amount and type of teacher-child interaction on child-child interaction during free play. *Psychology in the Schools*, 1976, *13*, 171–175.

Tilton, J., & Ottinger, D. Comparison of toy play behavior of autistic, retarded, and normal children. *Psychological Reports*, 1964, *15*, 967–975.

Wehman, P. Research on leisure time and the severely developmentally disabled. *Rehabilitation Literature*, 1977, *38*(4), 98–105.

Wehman, P. Effects of different environmental conditions on leisure time activity of the severely and profoundly handicapped. *Journal of Special Education*, 1978, *12*(2), 183–193.

Wehman, P. Toward a recreation curriculum for developmentally disabled persons. In: P. Wehman (Ed.), *Recreation Programming for Developmentally Disabled Persons*. Baltimore: University Park Press, 1979, 1–14.

Wehman, P. Teaching recreational skills to severely and profoundly handicapped persons. In: R. York & E. Edgar (Eds.), *Teaching the Severely Handicapped*, Vol. IV. Columbus, OH: Special Press, 1979.

Wehman, P., & Marchant, J. Developing gross motor recreation skills in children with severe behavioral handicaps. *Therapeutic Recreation Journal*, 1977, *11*(2), 48–54.

Wehman, P., & Marchant, J. Improving free play skills of severely retarded children. *American Journal of Occupational Therapy*, 1978, *32*(2), 100–104.

Wehman, P., Renzaglia, A., Berry, G., Schutz, R., & Karan, O. C. Developing a leisure skill repertoire in severely and profoundly handicapped adolescents and adults. *AAESPH Review*, 1978, *3*(3), 162–172.

Wehman, P., & Schleien, S. *Leisure skill curriculum for the developmentally disabled*. Working draft. Richmond, VA: School of Education, Virginia Commonwealth University, 1979.

Williams, W. W., & Fox, T. *Minimum Objective System*. Burlington, VT: University of Vermont, Center on Developmental Disabilities, 1977.

Williams, B., Briggs, N., & Williams, R. Selecting, adapting and understanding toys and recreation materials. In: P. Wehman (Ed.), *Recreation Programming for Developmentally Disabled Persons*. Baltimore: University Park Press, 1979, 15–36.

Chapter 3
LEISURE INSTRUCTION

The application of behavior modification techniques to the development of appropriate leisure activity in handicapped children and adults has increased in the past five years (Wehman, 1977; 1979). With the inclusion of recreation as a "related service" in the Education for Handicapped Children Act (PL 94-142), the implications are clear for special education teachers and therapists. Leisure skills must be assessed and taught to handicapped individuals. Recreational experiences should be provided that are chronologically age-appropriate and that help handicapped persons utilize their free time.

It is evident to many special education and recreation professionals, however, that recreational competencies do not always occur in handicapped individuals spontaneously. In fact, without systematically implemented programs that are based on the type of assessment procedures described in the previous chapter, recreational competencies will be limited. The ultimate goal of any leisure education program should be to facilitate self-initiated independent use of leisure time with chronologically age-appropriate recreational activities.

The purpose of this chapter, therefore, is to review the basic elements involved in the program development process when applied to leisure education. It is important that the reader understand the necessity of writing behavioral objectives, designing and utilizing task analyses, and implementing reinforcement procedures. These are the techniques upon which the leisure curriculum chapters, presented later in the text, are based.

PROGRAM DEVELOPMENT: WRITING BEHAVIORAL OBJECTIVES

Edginton and Hayes (1976) have stated the importance of writing behavioral objectives for a leisure education program. They stress the need for precision and accountability in recreational activities and suggest that instructional objectives are a critical aspect of program development. Public Law 94-142 also says that all Individual Education Plans (IEP's) should have clearly specified objectives.

Procedures for Specifying Instructional Objectives

According to Mager (1976), a behaviorally stated instructional objective involves three components: a statement of given conditions under which the desired performance should occur, a description of the desired performance, and a listing of the criterion for adequate performance. The program formats that provide the curricula in Chapter 6–9 each have an instructional objective as a guide for the therapist or teacher in program planning.

Specifying Performance Conditions The performance conditions specify the testing conditions (i.e., what the participant will be given or allowed to use during the testing situation). Such statements are usually introduced by the word "Given . . ." or "Using . . ." or "Referring to . . ." and the entire phrase generally precedes the terminal behavior. For example in a game of "Hand Slap," an objective might be:

> Given two participants, the participant will slap the top of his opponent's hands before the opponent moves his hands away 25% of the time.

Specifying Desired Performance When decisions are made about the desired performance, the enabling skills are selected in order to achieve the broad skill specified in the annual goals. Judgments should be based on what enabling skills the student has mastered and what enabling skills remain to be mastered before the broad skill is learned.

It is difficult to be explicit about the enabling skills the pupil must learn. The verbs that are used are the key element. These verbs must be concrete. Action skills are usually most descriptive; that is, they refer to unequivocal behavior that is clearly observable.

Specifying Criterion of Adequate Performance When the performance criterion is established, it is necessary to specify the *how well* part of the instructional objective. This is the achievement level that a teacher considers sufficient for the student to begin work on the next highest enabling skill. To specify the achievement level, it is necessary to decide about reference standards and cutting points.

Blake (1974) describes two types of reference standards: absolute mastery and relative mastery. Absolute mastery means criterion-referenced. Each individual's performance is judged against how much content is learned. The achievements of other individuals are immaterial. Relative mastery is norm-referenced. Each pupil's performance is judged against how much is learned in relation to how much other pupils learn.

After a reference standard is selected, the next decision is to identify the level of criterion expected. The question is: how much should the individual be expected to attain? At issue here is how much proficiency is required for enjoyment and participation. Total incompetence will inhibit participation. Complete mastery, on the other hand, may not be necessary. Criterion levels must be realistic as well. For example 100% criterion for making free throws in a basketball program would be highly unrealistic since professionals are rarely able to maintain this level of proficiency.

PROGRAM DEVELOPMENT: TASK ANALYSIS AND SKILL SEQUENCING

Once instructional objectives have been written, then the skill must be broken down into small components and logically sequenced. The order in which instructional objectives are presented greatly influences how handicapped individuals learn, which is the primary reason for the learning reliance on task analysis in Chapter 6-9. The amount of material that is presented will also influence learning (Blake, 1976). It is important that teachers and therapists develop instructional sequences that facilitate the use of these basic principles of learning.

Task analysis is the breaking down of skills into smaller components that may be easier for the individual to learn. It is a process that involves a logical sequencing of material from easy to more complex. A task analysis of an activity provides a precise description of the individual behaviors that are expected in a given recreational situation. For example, in most leisure programs, the therapist will ask a question or make a request of the individual in order to facilitate participation in a certain activity. The participant will in turn respond either correctly or incorrectly. Correct responses may be considered as target behaviors in a task analysis, i.e., step 1 or step 2 or step 6 in a task analysis format. Careful sequencing of the desired responses will ensure continuity within the program, as well as facilitate participation for the participator.

Skill sequencing may be considered as a logical progression of instructional objectives within a given domain. Williams and Gotts (1977) define a skill sequence as: ". . . delineated to provide a framework of tasks or objectives within which many types of instructional programs may be organized. A sequence is not a statement of how to teach but rather a statement of what is to be taught and in what order" (p. 221). A skill sequence is made up of several task analyses in a related area. For example, in a vending machine skill sequence, there might be a task analysis for *object identification, coin placement,* and *lever pulling.* Each of these skills would be taught separately to criterion and then eventually linked into a vending machine skill sequence. The continual development and field testing of reliable and valid skill sequences that are effective with handicapped individuals is an important task that faces special educators and recreation personnel.

What must be recognized, however, is that careful sequencing of skills is a critical aspect of the instructional situation between the teacher/ therapist and participant. Expensive materials, favorable staff ratios, and the most innovative of teaching activities are not being efficiently used when material is not presented in a logical sequence, or worse, when no sequence is provided at all.

The arbitrary selection of isolated leisure skills for handicapped individuals is an inadequate means of providing optimal leisure education.

In order for the individual educational program to flow logically and consistently over the approximately 18 years in school, skills selected from hobby, games, or sports domains must be clearly tied to the individual longitudinal or long-range educational needs.

THE NEED FOR TASK ANALYSIS COMPETENCIES

A task analysis approach to presenting information is optimal because it provides an instructional sequence and allows for the presentation of material in small chunks. By analyzing objectives into small increments that are logically sequenced, the participant will more quickly grasp the material. Special educators and therapists must be able to effectively employ task analyses and skill sequences in recreation programming and should thoroughly understand the multiple advantages of this approach. The efficiency of these techniques is validated in Chapter 10 with data collected daily on behavior change for several age-appropriate leisure activities, (i.e., darts), with severely multihandicapped adults.

Recent research clearly supports the efficacy of teaching in small chunks with more severely handicapped learners (e.g., Edgar, Maser, Smith, & Haring, 1977). With mildly handicapped individuals, the findings also indicate that in most cases the amount of material presented is directly related to the accuracy of the child's response (Blake, 1976).

Individualizing Instruction

A major advantage of a task analysis approach is that instruction for participants with different functioning levels may be individualized. Although some individuals may perform the majority of the steps or phases in a skill sequence, others will be unable to complete even one-third or one-fourth of the task. With task analysis, an individual's instructional program can be tailored to the appropriate functioning level. Furthermore, participants can move through the sequence at their own speed.

Homogeneous grouping within an activity plan, and according to skill level, may also be facilitated for each activity class. Because it is not usually realistic or practical to provide one-to-one instruction for each participant, it may be advantageous to place individuals in small groups with regard to their performance in a skill sequence.

Facilitating Teaching

In conducting precision assessments of the participant's given skill level in a given domain, it is helpful to pinpoint the entry level target behavior at which the person is presently functioning. With a task analysis it is possible to decide exactly where the participant requires assistance (Knapczyk, 1975). Reliable observational assessment will indicate strengths and weaknesses in a given leisure activity, thereby providing objective evidence that the individual needs a program prescribed to remediate those weaknesses. This specific assessment is done by the teacher as the participant's program is implemented.

Consider the following illustration of how an entry level skill in the motor domain might be assessed for a severely involved deaf-blind child. The specific skill of concern is standing up independently from a sitting position. For a profoundly deaf and blind child, sense of balance and equilibrium is grossly underdeveloped and requires training. In Table 1 is a task analysis for standing independently. Each "+" indicates that the step was performed with no assistance; "−" reveals that the child was unable to complete that part of the skill without physical assistance. It should be noted that this is only one possible task analysis of standing up behavior.

When this task analytic assessment is performed over a period of several days, it becomes apparent that there is a consistent breakdown in learning between steps 3 and 4. This suggests that the entry level to begin instruction is step 4. Finding behavioral pinpoints within well-developed instructional sequences facilitates learning by handicapped individuals and promotes more efficient instruction. Participants who receive instruction at a level in which they are already proficient will become bored; on the other hand, individuals who are taught component skills at too high a level are more likely to fail.

Objective Means of Evaluation

In order to evaluate progress that handicapped individuals make in leisure education programs, it is advantageous to objectively record the per-

Table 1. Task analysis for standing up

		Performs independently	Needs assistance
1.	Child sits on floor in four-point stance.	+	
2.	Child puts right foot flat on floor.	+	
3.	Child reaches for support table with right hand.	+	
4.	Child puts left foot on floor		
5.	Child straightens back and lifts head up.		−
6.	Child pulls self half-way up to standing position.		−
7.	Child pulls self three-quarter way up to standing position.		−
8.	Child stands up completely with support table.		−
9.	Child completes steps 4–8 without support table.		−

formance gains that are observed. Evaluating progress demonstrated on an instructional skill sequence is a logical extension of the assessment process described above. Use of task analysis sequences is one means of evaluation that will minimize teacher bias of the participant's progress.

One benefit of this form of evaluation is that it can provide reinforcing feedback to parents and teachers who are working with severely handicapped individuals. Students who exhibit gross language and motor handicaps usually progress very slowly. A task analysis sequence that is subdivided into minute behavioral increments will more precisely reflect the individual's progress. Although the steps achieved may be very small, it will still be positive to see the gains that can be made (Hanson, 1976; Mira, 1977).

Replicability

Another positive feature of a task analysis approach is that it facilitates replicability of the instructional program by other staff. If a skill sequence is implemented, there will be a logical order in which the participant's behavior should develop; there should also be a sequence to the behaviors that are required by the teacher in order to make the responses in the skill sequence occur.

In order for teaching associates, practicum students, student teachers, or other paraprofessional staff to effectively help the therapist carry through a program, there must be consistency. When the order of instructional behaviors is clearly specified, then, with minimal instruction, other staff should be able to implement the program. For substitute teachers who must fill in for extended periods of time, skill sequences are helpful.

It is also beneficial if other teachers can obtain similar results with instructional program sequences. If a certain task analysis facilitates learning for one activity class, it may be successful with another class. This might reduce the amount of time that educators must spend in selecting appropriately sequenced task analyses. Increasing success with selected task analyses will also suggest the empirical validity of such a sequence.

METHODS OF GENERATING SKILL SEQUENCES

To this point discussion has centered around why teachers should select relevant goals and objectives, and why task analysis is an important instructional competency. The purpose of this section is to identify and describe *how* to develop task analyses and skill sequences. Several specific methods of generating skill sequences and locating resources that facilitate the development of instructional sequences are delineated.

Reviewing Existing Resources

Once relevant leisure domains for instruction have been selected, it is necessary to do a careful review of the available commercial program literature. In recent years, more and more publishers have been providing texts that offer already completed and field-tested skill sequences. Through use of these books the teacher can save valuable curriculum development time by modifying, adapting, or replicating relevant instructional sequences.

A good example of one such resource is the text developed by Anderson, Hodson, and Jones (1974) entitled *Instructional Programming for the Handicapped Students*. Similar texts have been published by Bender and Valletutti (1976), and Myers, Sinco, and Stalma (1973).

The value of texts such as these is that replicable instructional sequences are provided that facilitate task-analytic assessment, learning in small parts, and objective evaluation. Furthermore, they usually span a large number of curricular areas across a wide range of disability categories; although the curricular areas do not always involve recreation, they are frequently related to maintaining participation in a variety of leisure activities. Clearly, the use of such commercial resources offers a savings in teacher time.

On the other hand, a cautionary note should be made. The wise teacher will not take every printed word as "the gospel"; it may be that some of the skill sequences that are published are inadequate or unacceptable. Simply because the work is published does not indicate that this is the only way, or even the right way. In selecting skill sequences from commercial resources, it is usually a good practice to confer with several other professionals involved in leisure programming with a similar population of students.

Modifying Developmental Sequences

Skill sequences may also be generated through careful perusal of textbooks that provide sequences of normal child development. In addition to child development texts, these sequences may be found in adaptive physical education books or occupational and physical therapy textbooks. Much of the cognitive-developmental theory generated by Jean Piaget (1962) may be helpful to the teacher in verifying whether curriculum content and sequence are relevant for students. Another excellent source of the sequencing of play cognitive development in infants is the work of Uzgiris and Hunt (1975).

Since most handicapped individuals are developmentally young in one or more curriculum areas, the application of child development norms to sequencing instructional content may be quite fruitful. Although developmental milestones are usually too broad for teachers to use as enabling skills, they provide a general developmental structure. This is particularly true in cases where little work has been published and is therefore not commercially available.

Adapting Curriculum Guides

Another means of identifying skill sequences that may be potentially useful is through careful inspection of curriculum guides that have relevant information. These include workbooks, detailed guides for a similar population of handicapped students, or "homemade" activity books developed by other teachers through experience.

In many ways, leisure materials and resources that are already available, although not exactly suitable for a given activity class, are an ideal source for therapists to review for skill sequences. They fulfill the criterion of being field-tested by other teachers. Frequently, such materials can be located quickly and inexpensively through the public school system or possibly a nearby university.

Breaking Down Skills Into Small Steps

In developing skill sequences, Williams (1975) has identified seven steps that must be carried through. These are listed below and are explained in detail.

1. Write the instructional objective for the enabling skill
2. Review instructional relevant resources for the task analysis breakdowns of the enabling skill
3. Derive the component skills of the objectives
4. Sequence the component skills
5. Eliminate unnecessary component skills
6. Eliminate redundant component skills
7. Determine prerequisite skills (p. 34)

Since writing an instructional objective was discussed in depth earlier, it is not necessary to further discuss this process. It should be apparent, however, that the instructional objective is the destination that the therapist is trying to help the participant reach. Following the skill sequence will move the individual closer to that objective.

As has been noted above, it is most efficient to review any possible resources that might be considered relevant to the task of generating a sequence. However, if this search proves fruitless, as it well may, particularly with the more severely involved student, then the component skills, or the basic steps of the task analysis, may be derived through several processes (Williams, 1975). Initially, it can be valuable to list all the components of a given skill that have been identified, although not sequenced, in other resources, such as curriculum guides and developmental scales. These components can then be arranged in an order that the activity therapist feels is a logical progression from easy to hard.

Another means of generating component skills for a task is to observe individuals and simply ask the question: "To master this objective, what skills must be performed?" This question is asked until further component skills cannot be performed.

A third process may also be effective. By slowly performing the target objective oneself or watching others complete the objective, one is able to record the skills that are necessary. Whether imagining the requisite skills or actually performing them, the teacher is sequentially taken through the skills that lead into the target objective. It is this precise type of task analysis that is necessary before goals of pinpoint assessment and evaluation, and learning in small steps can be accomplished.

Once the components of the target objective are identified through task analysis, then they must be arranged into the logical order required for completion. This process is usually done most effectively with input from several professionals. There are invariably several ways of presenting a skill. The majority of the task analyses generated in Chapters 6–9 are the product of input from occupational and physical therapists.

At this point it may be advantageous to review the sequence and determine whether there are any component skills within the sequence that are either not necessary or repetitious. Furthermore, it is best to "trialrun" the sequence initially before fully implementing it with the whole activity class. It may be that what seemed logical in the analysis stages is very clumsy for actual instructional purposes. It may also be that the skill has been subdivided so much that the "fun" is taken out of the activity.

In the final stage of development, core skills that are required to realistically perform the necessary component skills of the task must be identified. These skills can also be considered entry level skills or responses. Core skills are important because they indicate to the teacher at what level different participants must be performing before they can reasonably be expected to acquire the target objective. For example, in order to teach a deaf child to use sign language, a logical prerequisite skill would be motor imitation. A prerequisite skill to independent toileting might be proficiency in pulling down and pulling up pants. Considerably more discussion on core skills and how to use them in programming is provided in Chapter 5 on Curriculum Design.

PROGRAM DEVELOPMENT: TEACHING TECHNIQUES

Prompting, Fading, and Modeling

Three tactics of teaching new skills that have enjoyed much success are *prompting, fading,* and *modeling.* Frequently, handicapped persons either do not comprehend verbal instructions or do not comply with instructions. This is particularly characteristic of the moderately, severely, and profoundly retarded. When this occurs in a learning situation, the teacher or therapist is faced with how to get a desired behavior in an activity to occur. If the behavior is not demonstrated, little opportunity is present for reinforcement or for the client to realize the "fun" aspects of the activity. Only when the desired response is emitted and given positive reinforcement can the behavior become stronger.

When developing new leisure activities, a trainer may have to physically guide the individual through the desired activity. In order to encourage a profoundly retarded child to pull a wagon or roll a ball, the trainer may have to manually guide the child through the skill providing praise and affection contingent on successful approximations of the behavior.

Fading requires gradual removal of the physical guidance that is initially given in the development of the behavior. Timing the removal of the physical promptings is an art that a competent trainer gains only with experience; no amount of didactic instruction or lecture can replace the practical experience of prompting and fading. The importance of when to fade is critical. Removal of physical prompts too early or before the behavior is well-established will result in loss of the response, thus requiring that the response sequence be started again. Failure to fade a prompt, on the other hand, often leads to dependence on the trainer. It then becomes increasingly difficult to encourage independent behavior.

The aim of the competent therapist is to fade physical prompts to a simple gesture or pointing command, and eventually to achieve compliance with only verbal instructions. It is hoped that ultimately the individual's skill can be trained to a point where he behaves in accordance with environmental cues rather than instruction from the trainer.

In addition to prompting and fading as techniques, a therapist may also model an activity with the expectation that the observer will copy that behavior. When training disabled individuals who do not imitate readily, any modeled behavior that is matched by the subject should be reinforced immediately. The eventual goal demonstrated by researchers (e.g., Baer, Peterson, & Sherman, 1967) is to develop generalized imitation skills; that is, an ability to observe an activity and imitate it spontaneously.

Motor imitation is an effective form of communication that does not require verbal skills or constant physical guidance for learning. Acquisition of new skills may occur through vicarious learning and watching someone else in the environment.

Shaping and Chaining

The usual way in which a task analysis approach is implemented is through a behavior shaping procedure. With shaping, the terminal behavior objective is gained through reinforcing small steps or approximations toward the final response rather than reinforcing the final response itself. When developing new behavior, reinforcement may have to be given for approximations of the desired component skill. As the response becomes more accurate, reinforcement is only delivered for the correct response and previously reinforced approximations are ignored.

A sequence of responses in an activity may be referred to as a behavior chain. The game of "Hokey-Pokey" outlined in Table 2 is one example of a behavior chain. As Kazdin (1975) notes, "The component parts of a chain usually represent individual responses already in the repertoire of the individual. Yet the chain represents a combination of the individual responses ordered in a particular sequence" (p. 38). With this game the therapist trains the participant on the step he or she is unable to do. At the end of the instructional session, the participant is assisted through the *balance* of the skill. This is called forward chaining. *Backward chaining*, on the other hand, involves initially assisting the participant through all of the steps that the individual cannot complete. At the end of the chain instruction takes place. Hence if Stu, a severely retarded individual, cannot complete any of the steps in the "Hokey-Pokey" game, the therapist helps him through all of the steps except for Step 21. The same technique can be used for higher functioning individuals as well; the point of instruction, however, would be the last three to four steps, perhaps.

Cue Hierarchy

The basic instructional model that should be employed to implement the forward or backward chaining involves verbal instructions, modeling and gestures, and physical guidance. These techniques should follow a continuum of least drastic to most drastic. For example, selecting an item in a vending machine would be taught through application of the cue hierarchy in the following way:

Step One: Teacher provides verbal cue, i.e., "Tony, pull the lever." Praise is provided for correct response. Incorrect response leads to:

Step Two: Teacher repeats verbal cue plus models correct response, i.e., "Tony, pull the lever, like this . . ." (child must be attending to teacher). Praise is provided for correct response. Incorrect response leads to:

Step Three: Teacher repeats verbal cue plus physically guides Tony through steps he cannot do, i.e., "Tony, pull the lever." (Physical guidance provided.)

Once Tony has acquired all steps in the task analysis, then the teacher must remove the assistance gradually and also withdraw reinforcement

Table 2. "Hokey Pokey"

Instructional Objective: Given the song "Hokey Pokey" and a group of players arranged in a circle, the participant will sing and place his right foot, left foot, right hand, and left hand in the circle and take them out, and turn himself 360° while standing in place, at the appropriate times, 80% of the time.
Materials: "Hokey Pokey" record, record player, 4 or more players
Verbal Cue: "Diego, put your right foot in."

Task Analysis:
1. Stand in circle formation with other players, facing center of circle.
2. Attend to music and sing song, "You put your right foot in."
3. Bend at right knee lifting foot 6 inches off ground.
4. Move foot forward toward center of circle by extending at knee.
5. Place foot onto ground inside circle.
6. Sing song, "You take your right foot out."
7. Bend at right knee lifting foot 6 inches off ground.
8. Move foot backward away from center of circle.
9. Lower foot to ground onto perimeter of circle by extending at knee.
10. Sing song, "You put your right foot in and you shake it all about."
11. Place right foot inside circle again.
12. Rotate ankle from left to right to shake foot about.
13. Move foot backward away from center to normal standing position.
14. Sing song, "Do the Hokey Pokey and turn yourself about, that's what it's all about."
15. Turn body 1 complete revolution (360°) by pivoting on balls of feet to turn about.
16. Put left foot in circle.
17. Take left foot out.
18. Place left foot in and shake it about.
19. Do Hokey Pokey and turn body 360°.
20. Perform right hand movements.
21. Perform left hand movements to complete Hokey Pokey game.

Activity Guidelines/Special Adaptations
1. Teacher gives verbal cue to participant; if participant responds correctly, teacher provides reinforcement immediately.
2. If participant does not respond correctly, then teacher repeats verbal cue and models correct response.
3. If participant still does not respond correctly, then teacher repeats verbal cue and physically guides participant through correct response.
4. This instructional sequence is repeated several times in each training session with participant.
5. Participants could have their right arms and legs marked with colored ties to help identify appropriate limbs.
6. This musical game is an excellent means for teaching directionality, parts of the body and for improving gross motor skills and ability to follow directions.
7. Song and game can include several other motor movements using different body parts (i.e., chin, knee, backside, etc.).
8. With motor impaired individuals, use simple gross motor movements (i.e., place right ear in, requiring simple head turn).

slowly. The *fading* process is very important since the child must learn to perform independently.

This cue hierarchy is listed in each skill format within the curriculum. It should be done in conjunction with the other adaptations and techniques also described in this manual.

Selection and Use of Reinforcers

Reinforcer Sampling Frequently, teachers experience learning problems when developing programs for handicapped individuals. They do not know what to use for a reinforcer; they say the participant is unmotivated—he does not want to work for anything. At times, this may be a legitimate complaint. However, more often than not, the teacher has not exhausted the possibilities of developing novel reinforcers or has not utilized a reinforcer sampling technique (Ayllon & Azrin, 1968). Reinforcer sampling is the presenting of new types of stimuli and events to an individual and allowing him or her to explore or become familiar with these events. This increases the probability that the events will become reinforcing to the person.

Reinforcer sampling is most applicable to encouraging play and exploratory behavior in the retarded. Leisure materials are frequently strange stimuli with which a handicapped individual has not previously interacted. The reinforcing value of the materials has not been established; only through sampling different play materials will the child become aware of the reinforcing potential of the materials.

Reinforcement Menu A reinforcement event menu may consist of a large board with a number of high preference activities represented by stick figures or other symbols to indicate the different reinforcing activities available (Addison & Homme, 1966). This is one method of presenting a variety of reinforcer options to the child. It also has value because it can be observed and is not totally abstract. As Gardner (1974) notes, colored Polaroid® pictures or illustrations may be used to make the board more attractive and meaningful to younger children or the severely retarded individual.

Observation Many times, simple observation and trial-and-error method are used to determine the efficacy of reinforcing events with children. For several days the therapist may implement a certain reinforcement contingency on a desired behavior and evaluate if any behavior change is noted. Significant alterations in behavior may indicate that the reinforcer being employed is instrumental in the increase or decrease in behavior. This would be an example of the trial-and-error method.

Direct observation may also be used to effectively assess reinforcer preferences. Children who engage in certain activities or show great enthusiasm when given special privileges may work or demonstrate changed behavior if these events are made contingent on the desired behavior.

Usually, trial-and-error is used in combination with direct observation. Though it may appear that a child shows interest in certain activities or events, this does not necessarily mean that these events will effect a significant change in behavior. The teacher or therapist must systematically evaluate a range of reinforcing events and order them into a reinforcement hierarchy.

The Need for Specificity In determining reinforcing events, it is important to be specific. Each individual may respond differently under varied types of reinforcement. Social reinforcement may be too broad a term to describe the unique motivational conditions required for optimal performance.

Praise, physical affection, peer attention, or attention from different teachers are also possible combinations in which reinforcement may be delivered. It may be that an adolescent student works better during physical education period when the class is integrated with females. Certain individuals may perform under male reinforcement conditions rather than when a female is giving praise. These reinforcement variables may also be influential in determining the optimal motivational conditions in a behavior program.

Maximizing Reinforcer Effectiveness

Timing The immediacy of reinforcement is one variable that influences the efficacy of a reinforcer. Reinforcers need to be delivered contingent on the desired behavior, particularly when a response sequence is initially being developed. A child who begins to use toys in the play area should be immediately praised or given special attention. Similarly, a student who displays sharing behavior or cooperative play for the first time needs to be reinforced at once. Only in this way can the child gradually associate positive contingencies with the target behavior to be developed.

Labeling the Reinforcement Contingencies When a retarded person acts in an appropriate manner or begins to acquire a desired skill, the teacher must reinforce this behavior. However, it is critical that the individual be told *why* he or she is being reinforced. A common drawback of many leisure programs with the handicapped individual is the failure of a therapist to *label* the reinforcement contingency placed on the target behavior. For example, if cooperative play is encouraged between two children that frequently fight with each other, then any approximation of appropriate social interaction by either child should be rewarded with: "Good playing with Johnny!" and a pat on the back or hug. Severely handicapped students may not connect the positively reinforcing consequence with the desired behavior unless the contingency is labeled.

Amount of Reinforcement A general rule concerning magnitude of reinforcement is as follows: the greater the amount of reinforcement given for a response, the more frequent the response. This is true only to a certain point, however. If the magnitude of reinforcement is progressively increased, or is not varied with other reinforcers, then a reinforcer will lose its effect, causing satiation in the individual. Satiation may occur with any reinforcing stimuli or event, but is more likely to develop when primary reinforcers, i.e., food, liquid, are given excessively. Secondary reinforcers, such as praise or attention, are much more resistant to satiation effects.

It is probably best to use only social reinforcement for desired behavior unless responses will not develop without employing food or liquid reinforcers. In this way, the participant does not acquire a dependency on primary reinforcers, and learns to respond to the more natural reinforcements of praise and attention.

Schedule of Reinforcement A continuous schedule of reinforcement leads to the development of new behavior, while the gradual transition to an intermittent schedule promotes the maintenance or durability of the behavior pattern. Reinforcement is maximized in behavior development when reinforcers are delivered according to these reinforcement schedules. As a behavior becomes increasingly durable, the amount of reinforcement should be diminished, the delivery of reinforcers should become gradually delayed, and the schedule of reinforcement more intermittent.

The importance of identifying potent reinforcers and delivering them in a systematic fashion plays a large part in the development and success of an effective leisure program. Without careful use of the methods suggested, motivational conditions in the environment may not be appropriate for a desired level of performance or target behavior to occur.

PROGRAM DEVELOPMENT:
SKILL GENERALIZATION AND MAINTENANCE

The role of stimulus generalization, that is, learning to perform newly acquired skills in a variety of settings and situations, is an important area to avoid situation-specific learning. Below specific suggestions are advanced for facilitating transfer of training and maintenance of leisure skill proficiency.

Use of Naturally Occurring Reinforcers

Naturally occurring reinforcers are those events that are normal consequences of a behavior. Enjoyable leisure is a good illustration of a naturally occurring reinforcer once an individual has begun to acquire a leisure repertoire. As the individual's leisure behaviors increase, he becomes more aware of the pleasurable aspects of recreation and no longer needs special attention or privileges to maintain leisure behavior.

Alterations in Reinforcement Variables

There are several ways for maintaining leisure behaviors that have already been level through altering reinforcement variables. These are:

1. Fading the reinforcement contingencies gradually
2. Delaying the delivery of the reinforcer after a desired behavior occurs
3. Providing reinforcement on an intermittent schedule of reinforcement
4. Gradually reducing the amount of reinforcement given

It should be apparent that these methods are aimed to correspond closely to everyday reinforcement conditions under which most people live. While initially a learning situation for the handicapped may have to be structured and much more artificial for program results to be of any value, i.e., generalizable and durable, salient reinforcement variables must be modified as the child acquires the behavior.

Use of Parents and Peers

Transfer of training of program results may also be influenced through encouraging involvement in program planning and development from parents, relatives, siblings, and peers. Many programs originate in a setting away from home. Therefore, family knowledge and understanding of training procedures being utilized might be instrumental in generalizing the behavior into the home. One of the case studies in Chapter 10 describes the important role of parents.

Alternatively, parents are often able to give assistance to the teacher or trainer concerning their child's behavior at home. For instance, in developing a leisure program it is usually a good idea to get some initial direction from the child's home in toy preference, types or level of social interaction if any, length of time the child plays at one sitting, etc. This information may be modified and generalized to the classroom or activity class from the home.

Varying Stimulus Conditions

One of the more frequently used methods of promoting generalization has been to vary the stimulus (learning) conditions for training. This may include:

1. Introducing irrelevant or distracting stimuli
2. Utilizing a variety of teachers or trainers
3. Conducting the training in different settings

The aim of these procedures ". . . is to increase the number and type of stimuli which will set the occasion for the target behavior(s)" (Wehman, Abramson, & Norman, 1976, p. 2). It should be observed that the basic purpose of this form of generalization training is to help the child pick out the salient or critical components required to make the learning transfer.

These techniques were used to increase generalization of camera use by a multiply handicapped woman in a case study described in Chapter 10. In this program, the woman was taught how to use the camera and practiced with it at a local museum, park, and at home.

Some Practical Suggestions

In the Wehman, Abramson, and Norman (1976) paper, several implications were drawn from the literature review. These are summarized as follows:

1. Content should be selected with the consideration that it probably will play a role in the student's life away from the classroom.
2. Classroom teachers must gradually reduce the amount of reinforcement once the student has demonstrated the acquisition of a concept.
3. Students must practice newly acquired behaviors in a number of different settings and environments.
4. Classroom teachers must help the exceptional child establish his own reinforcer hierarchy.
5. Teachers must weigh the potential of peer control and the influence that peers can have on the durability of a behavior pattern.
6. Instructions given by teachers or peers should be explicit and, at least initially, followed by immediate behavioral consequences.

PROGRAM DEVELOPMENT: TRAINER COMPETENCIES

We now move from setting objectives, task analysis development, and program implementation to a delineation of the competencies that we feel therapeutic recreation specialists and special education teachers must have. If one divides leisure time into unstructured (free) activity versus structured (goal-oriented) activity, then a certain set of skills emerge that a therapist must demonstrate. These competencies, which are listed below, are based on the behavioral philosophy espoused in this book. They are necessary to understanding and implementing the curriculum in later chapters as well.

Unstructured Free Play

1. Given a free play situation with a number of objects available, a trainee performs a crude assessment of the developmental play level (i.e., autistic, isolative, or cooperative) of each participant.

2. Given a free play situation with a number of objects available, a trainee pairs instructions with modeling and demonstrates the function of the different toys of each child.
3. Given a free play situation with a number of objects available, in which the child does not respond to instructions and modeling, a trainee manually guides the child through playful action on different toys.
4. Given a free play situation with a number of objects and peers available, in which the child does not interact with peers, a trainee demonstrates proficiency in arranging interactions by (a) pairing a higher functioning peer model or adult model with the child or (b) pairing two isolated children together and serving as a mediator of social interaction between them.
5. Given a free play situation with children who are nonambulatory or who demonstrate little sensory awareness, a trainee demonstrates selection of objects that have a) configural complexity, b) sound potential, c) visual potential, or d) plasticity and that are durable.
6. Given a free play situation, a trainee demonstrates proficiency in constructing objects or adapting commercially available objects to the individual needs of the child.

Structured Leisure Activity

1. The trainee constructs skill sequences for a minimum of three community-based recreation programs and implements them with three handicapped adults.
2. The trainee constructs skill sequences for a minimum of three table games and card games and implements them with three handicapped children.
3. The trainee demonstrates to parents and families of a minimum of three handicapped children how to implement a table game skill sequence.
4. The trainee constructs and implements skill sequences and teaching sequences for a minimum of three group-oriented activities with a class of handicapped students.
5. The trainee constructs skill sequences in a minimum of three fine motor skill recreational activities and implements these sequences with three handicapped children.
6. The trainee constructs skill sequences with a minimum of three physical fitness exercises and implements these sequences with three handicapped adults.
7. The trainee constructs skill sequences with a minimum of five gross motor recreational activities and implements these sequences with five handicapped children or adults.

8. The trainee demonstrates proficiency across free activity and structured play situations in the following areas of reinforcement technique: a) selection of reinforcers, b) immediacy of reinforcement, c) selection of schedule of reinforcement, d) pairing of praise with affection and/or edibles, e) expressiveness of social reinforcement, and f) labeling of reinforcement contingency.
9. The trainee programs for transfer of training and response maintenance in free play and structured play situation by utilizing one of several of the strategies listed below:
   a. gradually fading out teacher assistance
   b. fading in higher functioning peers
   c. gradually reducing the amount of reinforcement
   d. teaching skills across environments

THE FINAL STEP: BEHAVIORAL EVALUATION OF THE PROGRAM

At least four questions must be asked and answered with a high degree of confidence when evaluating a program. The obvious first question lies in determining whether program objectives were met. If program results have been carefully monitored and the criterion met, this should be a relatively easy task.

The reliability of behavior observations must also be evaluated at this point. Results are of little value if based on erroneous observations of behavior. Also, at this time, the generalizability of newly developed leisure activities should be evaluated. Periodic followups of program results must be conducted to determine if the individual continues to engage in the activity independently.

The other primary evaluative component that deserves serious consideration is whether the procedures and/or adaptations employed to alter behavior were in fact responsible for behavior change, or whether outside uncontrolled sources influenced program results. This is important for use in future activity classes, and is best determined through employing an instructional design. An instructional design is a logical framework in which program results can be evaluated. While an involved discussion of research design is beyond the scope of this text, it is felt that a brief overview of basic instructional designs used in behavior modification may be beneficial.

Pretest-Teach-Posttest Design

One evaluation method used in many applied settings to compare before treatment and after treatment behavior is the pretest-teach-posttest design. First, a baseline or pretreatment measure of behavior is taken in the natural setting where the program is being conducted. When baseline responding is sufficiently stable, a treatment or intervention strategy is implemented. When a substantial behavior change is noted, a posttest measure of the target behavior is taken to evaluate extent of behavior change.

One example of this was observed in a recent play study with profoundly retarded children (Hopper & Wambold, 1976). The behavior being measured was frequency of appropriate play with toys; the intervention strategy was social reinforcement by teachers for appropriate play. In the pretest condition, low levels of responding were recorded for two of the children. However, after several weeks of treatment, a posttest evaluation indicated a substantial increase in the play behaviors of both children.

While the pretest-teach-posttest design is economical, easy to administer, and popular with many practitioners, it does have one serious drawback. Without a control group, that is, a group of similar subjects either randomly chosen or matched who do not receive the treatment, one cannot draw inferences that the intervention strategy was responsible for the behavior change. Other sources of variation in the environment (e.g., more attention at home, medication changes) could very well have contributed to the increase in play behaviors.

The Reversal Design

A more sophisticated method of evaluating efficacy of program procedures is a reversal design. In a reversal design, a target behavior is measured during a baseline period, and then an intervention strategy is implemented through use of a certain behavioral procedure. When a significant behavior change is noted, the behavioral procedure used to induce change is withdrawn. It is expected that responding will return to approximately the same level as during the first baseline period. When behavior drops to pretreatment level, the intervention strategy is employed once again to alter the behavior.

The logic behind a reversal design should be apparent. If a given behavioral procedure is responsible for increasing behavior and withdrawal of that procedure reduces behavior to its original level, then subsequent replications of the baseline-treatment sequence will lend additional support to the functional relationships between environmental manipulations and behavior change.

The reversal design is not usually employed in applied settings where little research is performed. Most practitioners do not care to withdraw reinforcement contingencies after laboring to develop a behavior in a client. However, from a research perspective, this is an excellent design for evaluating the efficacy of different instructional techniques or combinations of methods.

The Multiple Baseline Design

An alternative to a reversal design that is equally rigorous in evaluating experimental effects is the multiple baseline design (Hall, Cristler, Cranston, & Tucker, 1970; Kazdin, 1973). A multiple baseline design may be used across different types of behaviors, across different settings, and also across individuals.

When using a multiple baseline across different behaviors, baseline data are gathered on two or more independent behaviors. (See cooking case study in Chapter 10). After a stable responding rate is obtained, the intervention strategy is introduced with one of the behaviors. Data are continually gathered on both behaviors until a significant change is noted in the experimental condition. If responding on the other behavior has stayed at a continually low rate, the treatment is then utilized with the next behavior and changes in behavior are observed. This may be repeated across many behaviors to verify the efficacy of a given instructional method, and is valid as long as pretreatment baselines remain stable and do not change concomitantly with introduction of the treatment variable.

The strength of this design is that it allows for an experimental evaluation of the program results without disturbing the practical requirements of an applied setting. Greater use of multiple baseline designs is strongly advocated in behaviorally-based leisure education programs.

REFERENCES

Addison, R., & Homme, L. The reinforcing event (RE) menu. *National Society for Programmed Instruction Journal*, 1966, *5*, 8–9.

Anderson, R., Hodson, L., & Jones, R. *Instructional programming for handicapped students.* Springfield, IL: Charles C Thomas, 1974.

Ayllon, T., & Azrin, N. Reinforcer sampling: a technique for increasing the behavior of mental patients. *Journal of Applied Behavior Analysis*, 1968, *1*, 13–20.

Baer, D., Peterson, R., & Sherman, J. The development of imitation by reinforcing behavioral similarity to a model. *Journal of Experimental Analysis of Behavior*, 1967, *10*, 405–416.

Bender, M., & Valletutti, P. *Teaching the moderately and severely handicapped* (Vol. II). Baltimore: University Park Press, 1976.

Blake, K. A. *Teaching the retarded.* Englewood Cliffs, NJ: Prentice-Hall, 1974.

Blake, K. A. *The mentally retarded.* Englewood Cliffs, NJ: Prentice-Hall, 1976.

Edgar, E., Maser, J., Smith, D., & Haring, N. Developing an instructional sequence for teaching a self-help skill. *Education and Training of the Mentally Retarded*, 1977, *12*(1), 42–51.

Edginton, C., & Hayes, G. Using performance objectives in the delivery of therapeutic recreation services. *Leisurability*, 1976, *3*(4), 20–26.

Gardner, W. I. *Behavior management for children and youth.* Boston: Allyn and Bacon, 1974.

Hall, R. V., Cristler, C., Cranston, S., & Tucker, B. Teachers and parents as researchers using multiple baseline designs. *Journal of Applied Behavior Analysis*, 1970, *3*, 247–255.

Hanson, M. Evaluation of training procedures used in a parent implemented intervention program for Down's Syndrome infants. *AAESPH Review*, 1976, *1*(4), 36–55.

Hopper, D., & Wambold, C. An applied approach to improving the independent play behavior of severely mentally retarded children. *Education and Training of the Mentally Retarded*, 1976.

Kazdin, A. E. Methodological and assessment considerations in evaluating reinforcement programs in applied settings. *Journal of Applied Behavior Analysis*, 1973, *6*, 517–531.

Kazdin, A. E. *Behavior modification in applied settings.* Homewood, IL: Dorsey Press, 1975.

Knapzyk, D. Task analytic assessment for severe learning problems. *Education and Training of the Mentally Retarded.* 1975, *10*, 24–27.

Mager, R. *Preparing instructional objectives.* Belmont, CA: Fearon Publishers, 1976.

Mira, M. Tracking the motor behavior of multi-handicapped infants. *Mental Retardation*, 1977, *15*(3), 32–37.

Myers, D., Sinco, R., & Stalma, M. *The right-to-education child.* Springfield, IL: Charles C Thomas, 1973.

Piaget, J. *Play, dreams, and imitation.* New York: Norton, 1962.

Uzgiris, I., & Hunt, J. Mc V. *Instrument for assessing infant psychological development.* Urbana, IL: University of Illinois Press, 1975.

Wehman, P. *Helping the mentally retarded acquire play skills: A behavioral approach.* Springfield, IL: Charles C Thomas, 1977.

Wehman, P. (Ed.). *Recreation programming for developmentally disabled persons.* Baltimore: University Park Press, 1979.

Wehman, P., Abramson, M., & Norman, C. Transfer of training in behavior modification programs: An evaluative review. *Journal of Special Education*, 1977, *11*, 217–231.

Williams, W. W. Procedures of task analysis as related to developing instructional programs for severely handicapped students. In L. Brown, T. Crowner, W. Williams, & R. York. (Eds.), *Madison's alternative for zero exclusion* (Vol V). Madison, WI: Madison Public Schools, 1975.

Williams, W., & Gotts, E. Selected considerations on developing curriculum for severely handicapped students. In: E. Sontag, J. Smith, and N. Certo (Eds.) Educational Programming for the Severely and Profoundly Handicapped. Reston, VA: Council for Exceptional Children, 1977, pp. 221–226.

Chapter 4
ADAPTING LEISURE SKILLS

The various physical, social, and intellectual limitations of severely handicapped persons frequently prevent them from engaging in chronologically age-appropriate recreational activities. Disabilities act as barriers to participation, preventing individuals from constructively and creatively utilizing their free time. Many times it is necessary to modify activities to allow for full or partial participation.

An adaptation is a specific manipulation or change in any component of an activity. Every task contains several specifications for action. These may include the materials or equipment themselves, the manner in which the materials or equipment are manipulated, and any other environmental requirements necessary for performance. During leisure skill programming, adaptations can enable and even enhance a participant's performance. Socialization, self-sufficiency, motor development, and enjoyment are also facilitated. Ultimately, skill acquisition can lead to a more normalized life-style for the severely handicapped individual.

RATIONALE

By utilizing adaptations to simplify activities, barriers to participation can be eliminated. The removal of inhibitors can allow severely handicapped individuals to use recreational facilities, resources, materials, and equipment, thereby opening up various new experiences and avenues. Not only can participation be facilitated through the use of adaptations, but for many the experience of success can be obtained for the first time.

Not only are barriers to participation removed through appropriate implementation of adaptations, but attitude barriers can be overcome as well. Adaptations in various sports, games, and other socially related activities can allow a handicapped individual to participate with nonhandicapped peers. By participating in similar activities, increased acceptance in the home and community is facilitated. Instead of others in the environment observing and noticing the significant differences, interaction between the nonhandicapped and handicapped can create an awareness of their many similarities (O'Morrow, 1976). Once a limitation in a specific functioning area has been overcome through the use of adaptations, performance in other areas can be expressed to their full potential. For example, a cerebral palsied individual with an adapted playing card holder and shuffler could, for the first time, participate in a group card game and use his proficient communication skills. The adapted recreational activity becomes an excellent means of facilitating socialization, communication, and language skills.

Most severely handicapped persons require attention and special care in most aspects of daily living. Various modifications in the environment, however, can lead to greater independence. When applied to recreation, these adaptations allow the individual to exercise greater control over an abundance of leisure time. Freed from the need for constant assistance from others, the severely handicapped individual will gain an improved self-concept and greater sense of accomplishment. The acquisition of a leisure skill that now can be self-initiated and independently performed, enables the person to assume greater responsibility for his own life.

One of the principle difficulties in treatment of the severely handicapped is the time-consuming care, supervision, and prompting that must be offered because of their lack of self-initiated activity. The greater independence generated by a severely handicapped person's control of his own free time clearly reduces the need for constant custodial care. Greater autonomy can enhance the social relationships between staff and clients in the institution and among family members at home. With less time spent with the individual during his free time, staff members can devote more energy to more advanced and creative programming. Family members can pursue other areas of interest as well as have greater emotional freedom.

Recreation is also a vehicle by which gross and fine motor skills are developed. Inactivity usually results in poor eye-hand coordination, cardiovascular endurance, agility, dynamic and static balance, manual dexterity, and muscular strength. Because physical development is essential for a healthy body and self-concept, it is critical that severely handicapped persons be given every opportunity to experience recreation and develop physically. Frequently, only by adapting to simplify an activity, can the individual have the occasion to participate.

It has been noted that adapting a leisure skill can in some ways change the appearance of an activity. Consistent with the principle of normalization (Wolfensberger, 1972), all persons should learn and participate in as normal a manner as is feasible. Thus, the deleterious effects derived from adapting an activity must be taken into account. A modification should be used only when one is absolutely required. But the goal of any recreation program should be to allow the individual an opportunity to participate in a manner that will maximize the enjoyment obtained.

HISTORICAL BACKGROUND

For many years, equipment, supplies, and facilities have been adapted to meet the needs of the handicapped and disabled. The use of activity modification has been recorded in ancient societies dating as far back as

3000 B.C. In addition, adapted activities were used in schools for the deaf and blind in 18th century United States (Kraus, 1973). Recently, the use of such modifications has found its way into the fields of therapeutic recreation and special education.

Throughout the early part of the 20th century, recreation programs began to develop as an integral aspect of health care. The aftermath of World War II brought about a great need for specialized equipment and activity procedures. As disabled veterans returned home to the states, the development of organized recreation and specific programming expanded. Following World War II, recreation services that included the use of special adaptations became an integral component of rehabilitation and treatment. The Veterans Administration in 1945 established the Recreation Service as a part of its Hospital Special Services Division (O'Morrow, 1976).

Wheelchair sports developed from treatment programs at various veterans' hospitals across the United States. At the forefront of adapted activities, basketball arose as the most popular organized wheelchair sport. Within one year of the termination of the war, the Flying Wheels basketball team, composed of nonambulatory athletes, was already touring the United States (Adams, Daniel, & Rullman, 1975). The popularity of the adapted sport had far-reaching effects and facilitated the growth of adapted recreation for the handicapped.

As a result of the success of the wheelchair sports, recreation services in state institutions for the mentally ill were greatly accelerated. In 1948, Stoke Mandeville Hospital in Aylsburg, England introduced an organized wheelchair sports program for its patients. International games for the handicapped were first introduced at Stoke Mandeville Hospital in 1952. The United States, in 1960, entered international wheelchair competition for the first time. The Paralympics (Olympics for paraplegics) was held in the same year along with the Olympic games. Since that time, these games have taken place annually, and every fourth year they are held in the same city as the Olympic games. By 1960, lawn bowling, table tennis, javelin throwing, and swimming, among other sports, had been added to the ever-growing list of adapted recreation activities for the handicapped.

Recreation programs for the mentally retarded since World War II have also expanded. There is probably no hospital or institution in the United States today serving the mentally retarded that does not provide organized recreation (O'Morrow, 1976).

Considering the great strides made in the therapeutic recreation discipline since World War II, there has been comparatively minimal research activity concerning specific leisure-related adaptations. Through a review of the research literature concerning recreation programs for the handicapped, little can be found pertaining to the utilization and effectiveness of adaptations within the philosophy of therapeutic recreation. The following passages may provide some background regarding the use of adaptations and its place within the roles of rehabilitation and therapeutic recreation.

Modifying handicapped individuals' physical environments has been a concern of architects, therapists, and other professionals for many years (Goldsmith, 1963; Ries, 1973). Individuals and organizations have specified equipment and facility dimensions required for individuals with various disabilities. In Virginia, for example, the Commission of Outdoor Recreation recommends the following requirements for a public phone, which is certainly a leisure-related instrument. Telephone booths must have 32 inches clear entrance and telephones must be positioned so that the dial, receiver, and coin drop are no more than 4 feet above the floor.

In the 1950's, physical, occupational, and recreation therapists addressed themselves to finding ways of overcoming the barriers to recreation participation posed by the physical and intellectual deficiencies of the handicapped. Various basic modifications of recreational activity were devised, including equipment that allowed for the automatic return of a projectile to the player using tilted playing surfaces or by means of string or elastic attachments. In addition, researchers recommended the use of backstops and soft, flat projectiles that do not move or roll, thereby eliminating the need to retrieve the playing equipment. Consequently, modifications of this nature enhance the participation of many physically handicapped individuals in activities requiring large amounts of mobility.

Also in the 1950's, systematic studies concerning the need for and use of easy-to-handle sports and games equipment were performed. Hunt (1955) spoke of adapting activities and equipment for special populations. He offered a comprehensive philosophy concerning rehabilitation and recreation for the handicapped. He stated a responsibility for optimum development and opportunity to develop to the upper limits of each individual's capacities. Suggestions for specific implementation of this philosophy included the use of adaptations in equipment and procedure. Hunt recommended modified activities for the deaf, blind, orthopedically incapacitated, epileptic, mentally retarded, and other special groups.

Much of the work that transpired in the 1960's and 1970's consisted of presentations of rationales and philosophies related to the implementation of adaptations in recreational activities. Additionally, compilations of various material and procedural adaptations have been made. Special emphasis has been given to architectural design of leisure-related facilities. Fortunately for many individuals, state and federal legislation has facilitated such design considerations, thus eliminating architectural barriers.

Philosophies Concerning Adaptation Utilization
Many professionals agree that recreational activities, as well as skills in other curriculum areas, should be modified in such a manner as to promote normalization and mainstreaming (Tillman, 1973; Geddes & Burnette, 1975; Wehman, 1977; Brown, Branston-McClean, Baumgart, Vincent, Falvey, & Schroeder, 1979; Schleien & Kiernan, 1980).

Geddes and Burnette (1975) stated that adapting activities, when necessary, may allow handicapped persons to participate alongside their nonhandicapped peers, facilitating better integration into daily community activities. For example, an individual unable to play pinball, with the addition of an extended handle on the ball release knob and flippers, can participate in this table game at a community recreation center alongside his peers.

Adapting a recreational activity may also reduce institutionalization and promote mainstreaming into normal community living (Wehman, 1977; Schleien & Kiernan, 1980). The typical example occurs following the acquisition of a vocational skill by an individual in a sheltered workshop and the securing of a competitive job within the community. However, the hired person never acquired any recreational competencies or leisure skill repertoire. With an abundance of free, idle time in the evening hours, after returning home from work, and all day on weekends, this person returns to the institution for further training. Independent community living skills training, unfortunately, was not initially offered to the individual. With practical and creative recreational programming, along with modifications in the environment, the individual could become well-rounded and better able to cope with the unoccupied hours of each day.

Brown, a leader in the field of the education of the severely handicapped, and his associates (1979) addressed the need for partial participation utilizing adaptations, as opposed to no participation at all. They also mentioned that there is a critical need for varieties of adaptations that might allow or enhance participation.

It is obvious that by modifying an activity, the principles of normalization may be contradicted, that is the activity could become significantly different from its original version. In order for many of the goals of normalization to be reached, the programmer should be creative and inventive, when modifying activities (Tillman, 1973). For example, by analyzing an activity necessary adaptations can be more realistically and appropriately planned for because the actual participation requirements are already outlined. O'Morrow (1976) claims there are several components of every activity that can be considered (e.g., space required, number of participants, skill(s) required, etc.) before changing an original activity to its modified version. Gunn and Peterson (1978) developed an

Activity Analysis Rating Form by which a recreational activity can be evaluated in four behavior areas: physical, social, cognitive, and emotional/affective. Such an evaluation instrument can ensure that only necessary modifications commensurate with the participants' functioning level, capabilities, and needs are made.

Supporters of the human potential movement have espoused the use of activity modifications as a means of obtaining their goals. Earle and Yost (1975) state that all handicapped persons, including the deaf-blind, have the right to leisure activities and their benefits. Recreation professionals have the responsibility to provide for these individuals and to help them develop to their fullest capabilities. Through recreational activity, modified, simplified, or invented, handicapped persons are able to develop physically, socially, cognitively, and emotionally.

Conditions for Activity Modifications

There are several conditions under which an activity modification may be instituted. Gunn and Peterson (1978) identified two situations in which adaptations should be employed by the programmer. The first condition is when an individual is incapable of participating without an alteration in the original activity. A material or procedure may be modified for the sole purpose of allowing the individual to participate. The other condition calling for a special modification occurs within treatment or rehabilitation settings. In such an instance, activity analyses may determine that a specific adaptation could assist in attaining a treatment goal.

A number of professionals (Carlson & Ginglend, 1968; Thomas, 1974; Wehman & Schleien, 1979) have suggested a third instance warranting the use of a specific adaptation. Modified activities can act as leadup skills to the original sport, game, or hobby. Many times, the traditional activity is too demanding and/or intimidating for the individual. Initially, through the implementation of leadup skills, the potential participant engages in a similar, but simplified version of the original activity. This prepares him for eventual full participation in the targeted recreational pursuit.

Carlson and Ginglend (1968) discussed the implications of using leadup skills and activities to enable persons to learn and understand the smaller components of the larger individual or team sport. Some examples of modified leadup activities illustrated for the sport of baseball included: kickball for developing general concepts related to the playing field, scoring, and playing as a participating member of a team; and punchball to develop the gross motor coordination required. A description of 18 leadup activities adapted from the original sports were presented by Thomas (1974). An example given was newcomb and volleyball-modified as leadups for the game of volleyball.

The *Leisure Skills Curriculum for Developmentally Disabled Persons* (Wehman & Schleien, 1979) addresses the desirability of improving the readiness skills of the participant through leadup activities. This is the time when the person could practice and learn the fundamentals of the activity. "Solo Tennis," a game requiring the player to hit the tennis ball against a wall as many times as he can, is an excellent activity to practice the tennis stroke. With increased proficiency, he may begin to practice serving on an actual court. With the acquisition of these smaller skills, the player beomes prepared for tennis volleying with another person.

PROGRAMMATIC ADAPTATIONS

Programmatic adaptations of leisure activities may be considered a viable option for enhancing participation, especially for those persons with severe physical and/or sensory impairments. Because of the frequent need for skill simplification when working with this population, it is critical that the recreational programmer be knowledgeable in their appropriate and effective implementation. The remainder of this chapter addresses the when, what, and how of adapting leisure skills.

Guidelines to Consider When Adapting Leisure Skills

Many times, unfortunately, practitioners use adaptations without ever considering the needs of the participants. Frequently, the activity leader uses a material or procedural modification because it was purchased with funds difficult to come by, is presently available, or the teacher is familiar with its application. However, when using such criteria, the ability level of the participant is overlooked. A simplified version of the activity may not be required or necessary. He or she might successfully participate using the standard rules and equipment. A thorough activity analysis can pinpoint the facilitating, core, or prerequisite skills required for successful participation. Following the activity analysis, it is essential that the participant's ability to perform the requisite skills of the targeted activity be assessed. A modification should be applied only if it is positively essential for participation, success, and enjoyment. Adapt only when necessary!

An adaptation should be viewed as a temporary and transitional change in the original activity. Whenever possible, the leader and participant must work toward engagement in the original activity. The acquisition of a skill using modifications in one setting could become inapplicable and irrelevant in another. For instance, teaching the necessary skills for newcomb, a simplified version of volleyball, at the home agency would not be sufficient for participation in a mainstreamed community volleyball game. Newcomb requires the player to merely catch and throw the ball over the net. In a standard game of volleyball, however, the participant proficient only in the modified game would appear out of place on the playing court, thus becoming the butt of criticism rather than a candidate for normalization.

Because all severely handicapped persons function at different levels, adaptations must be made on an individual basis. An adapted physical education class was recently observed in which all twelve motorically handicapped students were tossing a lightweight Nerf frisbee. It was noted, however, that all but two of the students had the minimum eye-hand coordination required to throw a standard plastic frisbee. Nevertheless, when asked why all were using the modified equipment, the teacher responded, "We recently purchased a carton of Nerf frisbees for the school, and also it would probably be too dangerous for a few to be playing with a hard frisbee." Unfortunately for the remaining ten students, they never did receive instruction commensurate with their ability levels. The solution to this problem would have been to individualize the modification so that only the two pupils who needed to would use the special frisbee, while their classmates could learn to throw the more appropriate model.

If it is found that an individual does require a skill modification, care should be taken to keep the activity as close to the original or standard version as possible. The implementation of unnecessarily exaggerated adaptations can make the participant stand out by accentuating his disabilities. In this manner, others become more aware of the differences, and not the similarities between themselves and the "atypical" individual. Any necessary change in material or procedures should be made in order to maximize the benefits of normalization and mainstreaming.

So often an individual learns to use adapted equipment or materials exclusively at the home agency. However, the same modifications are usually not found or applicable in another setting. For example, a person who learns to bowl using a bowling ramp (See "Types of Recreational Adaptations—Material") may not be able to do so at a community alley where one is not available. It would seem that instruction in this case was for naught. It would have been more practical to teach the individual how to use a bowling ball pusher, which is less costly, portable, and therefore makes play accessible in any bowling alley. Admittedly, elaborate and expensive devices, such as the bowling ramp, are necessary for persons with more severe disabilities and should be employed. It is the therapist's/trainer's responsibility to consider several factors when making decisions of the sort described above. Cost, availability, and normalizing aspects of the modification must be studied. The first two considerations may sometimes be overcome by enterprising trainers who encourage community facility managers and owners to procure the specialized equipment themselves. Instead of feeling sorry for the handicapped, the business owner can purchase such devices as a wise business investment. A bowling alley owner who makes a bowling ramp available will consequently make his alley accessible to the handicapped citizens of the community. The resulting increase in patronage could very easily pay for the equipment many times over.

TYPES OF RECREATIONAL ADAPTATIONS

There are five types of adaptations that are considered here. They include 1) material adaptation, 2) rules or procedural adaptation, 3) skill sequence adaptation, 4) facility adaptation, and 5) leadup activity adaptations. Examples of each are presented below in leisure curriculum areas of games, sports, and hobbies.

Material Adaptations

Frequently, materials and equipment used in a recreational activity may act as barriers to participation. This is because the equipment commonly used during the activity was probably designed for nonhandicapped individuals and does not take into account the severe physical or sensory impairments of many severely handicapped persons. Therefore, it is often necessary to adapt or modify the equipment or materials thereby eliminating these barriers to recreation (Kraus, 1973).

As an illustration, consider the recreational needs of severely physically handicapped individuals who would like to bowl in a local bowling alley but lack the fine and gross motor coordination, balance, or muscular strength required to lift and roll a bowling ball down the alley. Fortunately, through material and/or equipment adaptations they overcome these difficulties. First, a tubular steel bowling ramp may be employed to allow nonambulatory individuals to participate. The ball is placed on top of the ramp and the bowler must then simply position the ramp toward the desired pins and release the ball. Second, a bowling ball pusher may also be used to enhance participation. It is designed to push the ball down the alley like a shuffleboard stick. The pusher can be adjusted to various lengths allowing both ambulatory, nonambulatory, short and tall individuals to play. A third adapted device that can be used by a person unable to lift a conventional ball is a handle grip bowling ball. It only requires a simple palmar grasp and basic gross motor arm movements to manipulate. Once released, the handle snaps back flush into the bowling ball, allowing the ball to roll toward the pins. It is obvious that with all the adapted bowling equipment available, many physically handicapped persons can bowl and enjoy the sport. Figures 1, 2, and 3 provide illustrations of each of these devices.

A plethora of specialized equipment for the quadriplegic patient was described by Ford and Duckworth (1976). They addressed the issue of

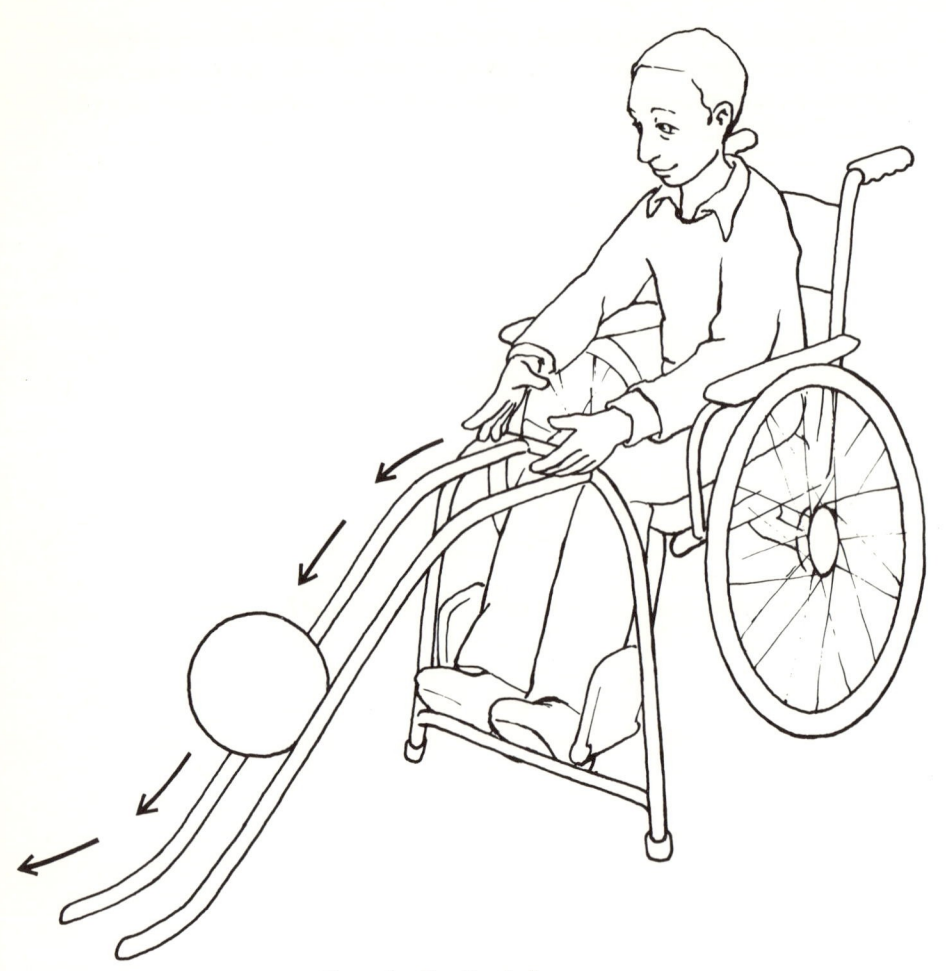

Figure 1. Bowling ball ramp.

recreational adaptations, such as the use of a special splint to help pull back the bow string in the sport of archery. A stand that holds a telephone receiver in the appropriate speaking position for the person who cannot hold a receiver was illustrated. Several useful tips and modified devices for cooking, reading, playing cards, and cutting with scissors were also presented.

Sherman (1975), in working with young blind and deaf-blind children at Washington State School for the Blind, discovered the difficulties in capturing the interest of many of these children and in awakening curiosity and awareness of their surroundings. By adapting materials to simplify the manipulatory responses required, she was able to develop and stimulate interest in several blind students. Sherman devised a handicrafts program encompassing a wide variety of learning experiences and recommended various types of adapted equipment to simplify recreational activities for this special population. She described dual scissors (4 hole

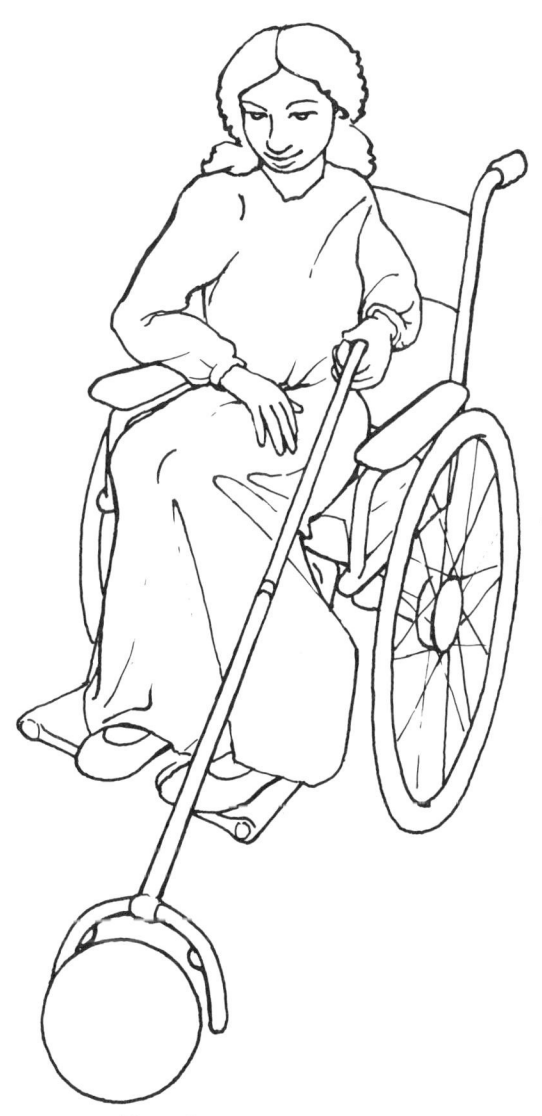

Figure 2. Bowling ball pusher.

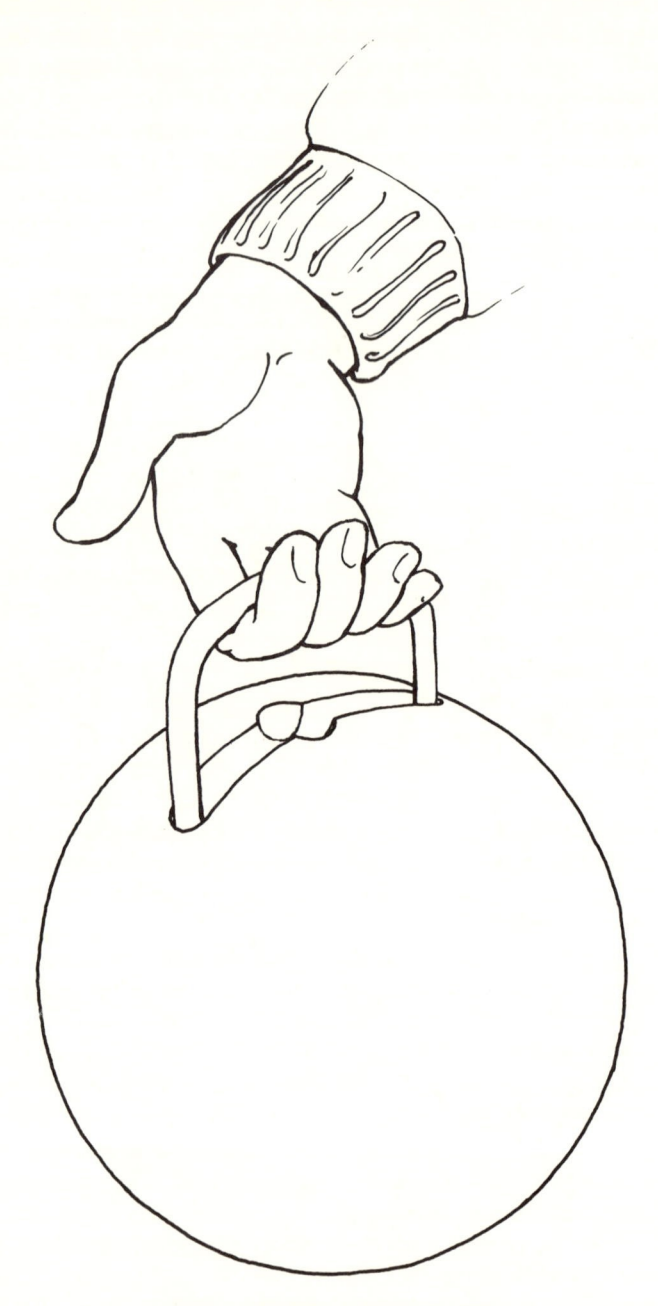

Figure 3. Handle grip bowling ball.

training scissors) as an excellent device for teaching cutting. By riding piggyback on the student's hand, the teacher can help the participant go through the motions for working the scissors. Sherman also described sewing modifications. Stringing beads is the first step, to be followed by giving the blind person yarn on a blunt needle and a piece of plastic window screening. The student should be allowed to stitch at random to learn what the yarn and needle can do. Sherman concluded with a compilation of leisure-related equipment for the blind and where to find them. A few of the adapted materials mentioned were a crockpot cookbook, greeting cards, paper money identifiers, and sewing machine.

According to Earle and Yost (1975), by means of modified, simplified, or invented recreational activity, deaf-blind individuals are able to develop leisure repertoires, experience success and failures, improve coordination, and develop skills of problem solving and creativity. The authors continue to list several adapted sports activities that are appropriate, rewarding, fun, and have been successful with this population. They describe the necessary equipment adaptations, but insist that activities requiring few changes are desirable since they represent the normal activity. They recommend a beeping target in archery for those with a degree of hearing. A stick used for a guide to assist the archer with lining up his bow and arrow is also explained.

Adams, Daniel, and Rullman (1975) also discussed ways of adapting the materials involved in games, sports, and exercises. Modifications were presented making activities accessible to people with various handicapping conditions (e.g., blind, cerebral palsy, obesity, amputee, paraplegic, etc.). For each activity, disabilities were identified along with their respective adaptation suggestions. Such a presentation of special adaptations represents a boon to the programmer. With this material, he can more efficiently individualize the recreation program to meet the specific needs of the participants. For instance, a blind bowler may require a guide rail to assist in aiming the ball down the alley, whereas a bowling ramp may be a necessary adaptation for a player with cerebral palsy. Another example cited was the use of a bi-handled paddle to allow an arthritic participant to play ping pong. Such an adapted piece of equipment permits easier manipulation of the paddle when hand joints are seriously involved. For an individual suffering from malnutritional weakness, playing ping pong from a wheelchair was the suggested adaptation. Adapted group and individualized activities were discussed along with design diagrams of specialized equipment.

Many types of special equipment are commercially available and can be purchased from sporting goods and hobby stores, specialty shops, and mail order houses. However, budgeting factors and the skyrocketing price increases of most commercially available equipment have made a need for inexpensive recreational materials and adapted equipment that can be constructed by the teacher or therapist.

The American Alliance for Health, Physical Education, and Recreation (1977) listed and described 29 pieces of equipment and devices used by handicapped persons to permit full participation in various physical activities. Equipment, devices for ball activities, bowling aids, and assistive devices for young children were presented. For each piece of equipment a homemade alternative was described along with information concerning the availability of commercially marketed items. An example is the homemade and less expensive alternative to the Schwimmfugel. The commercially available Schwimmfugel consists of inflatable cuffs that are worn around the arms to keep the nonswimmer afloat. Instead, empty bottles tied around the arms with pieces of fabric make a functional substitute. Another successful teachermade sporting goods adaptation is an enlarged tennis racket handle. Sponge or foam rubber wrapped with masking tape allows for easier grasping and control.

Homemade equipment and other adaptable ideas that make it possible for handicapped students to participate, to some degree, in several popular gross motor sporting activities have been discussed. Cowart (1973) presented a spotting device for a weightlifting bench press. The device was constructed to support the weight of the barbell while not in actual use. It prevents the weightlifter from being hit with the weights if accidentally dropped during the lifting process and acts as a guide for the barbell during the lift. Cowart contends that the teacher is confronted with students having a wide variety of physical problems. Equipment and supplies are occasionally not available in the schools to meet the students' needs. But with a little time, initiative, and creativity, many items can be made inexpensively. Additionally, existing equipment can be adapted to enhance participation and success. To meet specific individual needs, the author described items that have been developed and equipment that has been adjusted. As a consequence, individuals formerly unable to participate have found new opportunities commensurate with their capabilities.

A booklet written by the Florida Learning Resources System (1976) provides descriptions of several teachermade recreational activities for use with handicapped children. One game described called "Comic Strips" consists of related pictures that must be put in correct sequential order by the participant. Information relating to each game including objectives, target population, materials, and procedures were offered.

Lear (1977) described a number of specialized toys and activities for handicapped children that could be made by teachers and parents. Most of the toys presented could be constructed from common items. An example of a modified sewing activity was presented that uses a piece of cardboard as a base. Lear suggested drawing the illustration on both sides of the card and punching holes where the stitches must go. These two modifications of material simplify the sewing task because, by drawing a picture on the back of the cards as well, it is easier for the person to determine the location of the following stitch.

The myriad of commercially available and homemade material adaptations aid in the elimination of barriers to participation and make a number of chronologically age-appropriate enjoyable activities accessible to all those who wish to participate. Mason (1969) discovered that with the implementation of special equipment, individuals with almost any handicapping condition could participate and compete alongside their normal peers. Consequences for normalization are suggested. At the same time, special modifications eliminate the use of age-inappropriate recreational materials that, in the past, might have been the individual's only alternative. Other examples of material adaptations are illustrated in Table 1.

Procedural/Rule Adaptations

Just as materials and equipment can act as barriers to participation, so may the procedures and rules of a recreational activity. Most games or activities contain a standard set of rules that must be followed. If a rule makes an activity too difficult for a handicapped individual, it may result in the potential participant becoming a spectator. These difficulties need not be insurmountable. They may be overcome by increased use of changes in the original rules of activities.

For example, the standard game of basketball requires a player to bounce or dribble the ball every time he takes a step. Through a simple rule change that allows for one dribble for several steps down the court, an individual possessing inadequate eye-hand coordination can now become an active member of the team. Additionally, persons confined to wheelchairs can now participate and compete in basketball play by altering rules and procedures. The National Wheelchair Basketball Association developed the following rules and regulations for wheelchair basketball play:

> *RULES AND REGULATIONS* for wheelchair basketball are the same as the national basketball rules *except* for the following changes.
> 1. The rear wheels are on the free-throw line for free throws.
> 2. A player is not allowed to hold, push, or intentionally contact another player's wheelchair. Time is called if a player falls out of his wheelchair.
> 3. A player is allowed only 15 seconds to advance the ball from the back to the front of the court. He is allowed only 6 seconds in the free-throw circle when in possession of the ball.
> 4. Players must remain seated in their wheelchairs. When in possession of the ball, a player must push the wheels of his chair only twice until he bounces the ball twice on the floor or passes (Hunt, 1955).

Table 1. Material adaptations for leisure skills

Standard skill	Easier/modified skill
1. Inflating balloon	1. Use of cardboard pump to inflate balloon
2. Camera skill: manipulation of shutter release button and general operation	2. a. Extend button with wax crayon attachment b. Color designated buttons
3. Crayon drawing	3. a. Enlarged crayons b. Use of wooden crayon holder
4. Hold flashlight	4. Attach flashlight to velcro wristlet
5. Toss regulation plastic frisbee	5. Throw lightweight Nerf frisbee
6. Cut with scissors	6. a. Use four-holed training scissors b. Use blunt scissors for safety
7. Use of telephone	7. a. Designate receiving and sending end of receiver with pictures of ear and mouth b. Push button telephone c. Receiver shoulder rest d. Stationary receiver-holding stand
8. Tic-Tac-Toe: pencil and paper version	8. Tic-Tac-Toe board game with easy to grasp enlarged X's and O's
9. Badminton: standard racket outdoor play regulation net standard birdie	9. a. Short-handled racket b. Enlarged foam rubber racket handle c. Indoor play (eliminate wind factor) d. Lowered net e. Lightweight (ball or yarn) or heavier weighted birdie
10. Basketball	10. a. Smaller or larger ball (multipurpose ball, etc.) b. Lower basketball backboard c. Larger basketball hoop d. Controlled basketball unit (returns ball to wheelchairbound participant) e. Use of paddle to dribble ball f. Nerf basketball
11. Bowling	11. a. Tubular steel bowling ramp b. Bowling ball pusher c. Handle grip bowling ball d. Nerf ball with holes e. Guiderail (for blind bowlers)
12. Sleeping bag: camping	12. Extended zipper (easier to grasp)
13. Cooking: pour liquid cooking utensils oven use	13. a. Container with pouring spout (easier pouring for individuals with poor motor coordination) b. Utensil handles can be enlarged using tape and foam rubber c. Color-coded dials for top burners and oven d. Tape strips for easily distinguishable dial and timer calibrations

To enhance participation in a wide variety of activities, Thomas (1974) outlined a number of procedurally modified exercises to provide physical activity for wheelchair patients. He claimed the exercises serve a dual purpose: to increase strength, flexibility, endurance, and agility, and to provide a learning, movement experience. Modified exercises addressed included: pushups to increase strength in the upper extremeties and shoulder girdle; leg lifts (quad setting) to increase strength and flexibility of the legs, especially the quadriceps muscles and the muscles of the lower pelvic girdle; toe touches to increase strength and flexibility of the lower back and shoulder girdle; wheelchair situps to strengthen the lower back; and front and rear wall pushes to develop an increased strength and flexibility in the arm and shoulder girdle associated with moving the wheelchair forward and in reverse.

In 1975, Amary described a number of games for the nonambulatory mentally retarded person. Among other innovations, the procedures necessary for wheelchair badminton and relay races were outlined. As an example, the author's variation to regular badminton allows each player to hit the shuttlecock twice before it is passed on.

The Information and Research Utilization Center in Physical Education and Recreation for the Handicapped (1976) compiled a series of booklets discussing recreation and physical education activities and teaching strategies for the handicapped. Their goal was to stimulate and encourage programmers to adapt activities and attempt new and creative approaches. Specific activity modifications for individuals with varying degrees and types of conditions were outlined. The booklet contains methods, equipment needs, adaptations, and physical layouts required for activity simplification. Their suggestions for procedural adaptations in a special volleyball game included: allowing the participant to throw the ball over the net for a serve or serving closer to the net and allowing the participant to catch and throw the ball over the net rather than hit and volley it.

Billiards or pool can also be made more accessible to a person who is unable to identify the striped or solid balls during a game of 8-ball. This problem may arise due to a sensory or perceptual deficit. Rather than designating certain balls to specific participants, the game can consist of participants taking turns and shooting at any ball on the table. The number of balls hit into the pocket is recorded and the individual with the most balls pocketed declared the winner.

There are a wide variety of card games that are appropriate to adults. One such game is Concentration. This game requires the player to draw two cards consecutively, the object being to draw the greatest number of pairs. For many severely handicapped individuals the picture cards present a problem in discrimination. A procedural adaptation that allows such a person to participate makes all pictures (i.e., jacks, queens, kings) the same value. In this manner, an individual would only have to discriminate between numbered and pictured cards. Additionally, the ace card could be modified by whiting out the symbol "A" and replacing it with the number "1."

Modifications in procedures and rules can turn a seemingly impossible task into an enjoyable recreational pursuit. Changing the rules of a complex activity may allow an adolescent or adult to participate in an age-appropriate game or sport. This strategy is more normalizing than having the individual resort to the manipulation of an age-inappropriate toy or youngster's game. See Table 2 for additional procedural/rule adaptations.

Skill Sequence Adaptations

One of the most effective ways to teach a severely handicapped individual a recreational activity is to break the skill down into smaller component steps (Wehman and Schleien, 1979). These actions are identified through an analysis of the task itself and are subsequently sequenced in a logical order. However, a sequence of steps applicable to a nonhandicapped individual often may prove too difficult or impractical for a severely handicapped person to follow.

A hobby such as cooking can provide a clear illustration of the problem. When boiling an egg, a nonhandicapped person might place the egg into a pot of boiling water. It is obvious that this could be a hazardous problem (i.e., scald hand) for an individual with physical and/or intellec-

Table 2. Procedural/rule adaptations for leisure skills

Standard skill	Easier/modified skill
1. Badminton	1. Stand closer to net (3 feet) to ensure more proficient shot
2. Basketball	2. a. More than 5 players (increase court coverage and eliminate need for long passes) b. Use half a court c. Allow two-handed dribbling d. Allow two or more steps per dribble
3. Bowling	3. Allow individual to stand closer to pins (beyond foul line)
4. Carrom board game	4. Use fingers instead of cue stick to flick carroms across board (for one-handed play)
5. Billiards: 8-ball	5. Rather than designate striped or solid balls, shoot at any ball and record number of balls hit into pockets
6. Concentration card game	6. All picture cards (jack, queen, king) possess same value

tual limitations. A remedy to this problem is to rearrange the sequence of the component steps of the skill by training the cook to initially place the egg into the saucepan and then filling the pot with cold water. The saucepan is then placed onto the top stove burner and the water brought to a boil. This procedure does not alter the final results (i.e., boiled egg), but does facilitate a safe and practical method of performing this worthwhile leisure pursuit.

A modified skill sequence applicable to the manipulation of a camera can also be implemented. Typically, an individual will first raise the camera to eye level and then place his index finger over the shutter release button. However, individuals lacking sufficient fine motor coordination can initially be trained to position their finger over the shutter release button prior to lifting the camera. In this way, the individual would merely have to depress the button once the camera was appropriately positioned.

The use of a task analysis is an important tool in the programming of leisure skills for the severely handicapped individual. But at times, the teacher or trainer may find it necessary to alter the normal chain of behaviors involved so the participant may succeed and more readily gain satisfaction from the activity. Other skill sequence modifications are identified in Table 3.

Community-Based Facility Adaptations

The community itself offers many age-appropriate recreational avenues of which nonhandicapped individuals regularly take advantage. A local swimming pool, museum, restaurant, library, or church are all public facilities available to handicapped people. Unfortunately, many severely handicapped individuals are denied access to these places and subsequently cannot utilize their leisure time in these environments. This problem is most evident for nonambulatory individuals who are unable to enter public buildings because of narrow doors, inadequate toilet facilities, and imposing staircases. In addition, transportation to many of these facilities in inadequate.

However, many of these architectural barriers have been and can be overcome by the installation of wheelchair ramps leading to buildings, enlarged doorknobs, extended handles on drinking fountains, and other adapted equipment that aids those with severe motor impairments.

Federal and state legislation has been passed with the intent of increasing the accessibility of public buildings and facilities for all. In 1973, Section 504 of the Vocational Rehabilitation Act was passed to meet this goal. The state of Virginia's Commission of Outdoor Recreation (1976) has set guidelines to assist with the elimination of architectural barriers. Special parking areas, wheelchair ramps, curb cuts, and other necessary facility modifications were recommended. Specifications were set for

Table 3. Skill sequence adaptations for leisure skills

Standard skill	Easier/modified skill
1. Boil egg: place egg into saucepan of boiling water	1. Place egg into saucepan filled with cold water, then boil (safety factor)
2. Camera skill: raise camera to eye level, then position finger on shutter release button	2. Position finger on shutter release button, then raise camera to eye level
3. Card game: pick up each playing card one-by-one, as dealt	3. "Dealers courtesy"—pick up playing cards only after all have been dealt to all players (for easier manipulation)
4. Beach trip: dress at bath house	4. Dress in swim attire before leaving home (easier to dress in familiar environment)
5. Fast foods restaurant: order meal immediately upon entering	5. Procure menu initially so that meal selection is accomplished prior to entering restaurant (less pressured environment and allows more time to make decisions)
6. Make telephone call from public booth: take money out of pants pocket after receiver is properly positioned against ear and mouth	6. Place correct change on counter before picking up receiver
7. Cooking: preheat oven before placing food in oven	7. Place food in oven before turning oven on (safety factor)
8. General preparation of food: take items from refrigerator and cabinets when needed	8. Have all necessary food items in view and within reach before beginning to combine ingredients

facilities such as elevators, drinking fountains, and public restrooms. Among the modifications required for parking lots at parks and recreational facilities are covers on drains in driveways so that wheelchair mobility is not impeded. Wheelchair access to drive-up phones and specifications for parking spaces consisted of clearly identified 12 feet 6-inch minimum width slots for handicapped persons located near facility entrances. It was required that two spaces be available for the handicapped for every 20 spaces in each lot.

Legislation is presently being passed that requires all telephone areas for public use to contain at least one telephone that can be used by the physically disabled. Telephone booths should be avoided in favor of the open telephone station. In Virginia, for example, the Commission recommended the following requirements for public phones: telephone booths must have a 32-inch clear entrance; telephones must be placed so that the dial, receiver, and coin drop are no more than 4 feet above the floor. In addition, push button telephones are rapidly replacing the older models, eliminating the need to dial in a circular clockwise fashion. Receivers are becoming equipped with adjustable audio control devices that increase volume for those with hearing deficiencies.

The Commission made the following suggestions concerning community sporting facilities to accommodate the disabled: basketball goals and backdrops should be available from heights of 6 to 10 feet in 1-foot increments; all game areas should be enclosed within fences to keep balls and other equipment from leaving the play area; outdoor carpet over hard surfaces can aid in golf putting; devices to retrieve golf balls should be placed in holes and ends of golfing greens; greens should be 4 feet wide to allow a wheelchair to reach the hole. (It is interesting to note that, although miniature golf has been popular among the general population for years, it was not until 1967 that an adapted regulation miniature golf course was designed for the handicapped. The Children's Rehabilitation Center at the University of Virginia led the way in the development of this adapted sport (Adams, Daniel, & Rullman, 1975). Table tennis, football, and other table sports can be accessible to wheelchair users if adequate clear space for movement is provided. Generally, at least 5 feet should be allowed between the edge of the table and the nearest wall, table, or other areas. Also included in the Commission's manual are guidelines for: vehicular and pedestrian circulation, other recreation facilities, childrens' play areas, buildings and utilities, and furnishings (e.g., benches, tables, grills, water fountains, campfires).

Architects, professional organizations, and recreation professionals have also suggested ways of making facilities more accessible. Ries (1973) presented a manual of design standards for the physically handicapped. Specifications for equipment and facilities were discussed, and diagrammed illustrations were also included. Examples relevant to recreation include: adapted swimming facilities (special walkway dimensions, guide bars, and sloping ramps leading into the water), modified basketball courts (lower backboard, fenced enclosure), and adapted public telephones (easy access booths, lower to ground).

Goldsmith (1963) prepared a manual covering various aspects of building design relevant to the disabled. The public and domestic facility design modifications addressed all aspects of the architectural environment including leisure-related areas such as cooking facilities. Goldsmith's recommendations for kitchen design emphasized ease of movement between the principal working areas and accessibility to appliances. Additionally, the author supported the rehabilitation and reintegration of disabled persons into society whenever possible. In order to attain this goal, provisions were made for modifying public facilities to allow for greater utilization by the handicapped.

The American Alliance for Health, Physical Education, and Recreation (1977) published a document dealing with a wide variety of means to overcome architectural and facility barriers through the use of adaptations. The populations for which these modifications are geared include the physically impaired and those with orthopedic conditions. Lists of adapted material and design guidelines were presented. The bibliography contains an outline of selected laws pertaining to architectural accessibility and a listing of relevant journals addressing similar legislation.

Nesbitt (1970) concentrated his efforts on community-based recreational areas and facilities for the economically disadvantaged within the inner city. Modifications for various aspects of recreation environments, including cultural, transportation, and equipment were discussed.

A general outline for adapting public facilities is given by Kraus (1973), a leader in the field of therapeutic recreation. He encourages the use of paths and ramps for wheelchairs, wider and easier to open doorways, grab bars in restrooms, lowered drinking fountains, and many other considerations in architectural design.

While these physical modifications are reducing barriers to utilization, there is one principle that must be seriously considered. The person utilizing the equipment or facility must not, at the same time, be separated from interacting with the community in general. The environmental modifications must be as normalizing as possible, making sure not to isolate the handicapped individual. Brown, et al. (1979) summarized that it is just as important to plan for the severely handicapped's social, emotional, educational, and other needs as it is for physical accessibility. For example, they suggested that adapted playground equipment need not be isolated from the remaining playground facilities. Means for socializing and other needs of the individual should be enhanced rather than stifled by the use of gross facility modifications. Pier fishing could be made accessible to physically impaired individuals and retain its normal qualities. Guidelines require: an access walk to the pier of at least a 5-foot width to allow for turning of the wheelchairs; the provision of a handrail around the entire pier that, according to the Virginia Commission of Outdoor Recreation, must be 36 inches high and have a 30° angle sloping top for arm and pole rest; a kick plate to prevent foot pedals of wheelchairs from going off the pier; and finally, a smooth, nonslip surface should be provided on the access walk as well as on the pier.

All activities enjoyed by the nonhandicapped can be experienced by disabled persons as well. Equipment and facility modifications can often be minimal and implemented for a reasonable cost (Pomeroy, 1964). Presently, the task at hand involves the alteration of already existing facilities. The task for present and future planners is to incorporate these necessary facility specifications into community recreational developments. If such modifications are made at inception, costs for adapting facilities could be kept to a minimum. For additional community-based facility adaptations, refer to Table 4.

Leadup Activity Adaptations

A leadup activity is a simplified version of a traditional activity or an exercise that allows for practice in some component skill of a game, sport,

Table 4. Community based facility adaptations for leisure skills

Standard facility	Modified facility
1. Community swimming pool	1. a. Built up pool ridges (reduced chance of falling into pool accidentally)
	b. Steps leading into pool with handrails should have short tiers and wide steps
	c. Ropes and floating corks to divide deepest from shallow ends and as a guiderail to ladders
	d. Hydraulic lift for pool entrance for nonambulatory persons
	e. Protrusions on pool bottom to mark shallow end and direct swimmer to ladder
	f. Nonslip and nonabrasive pool and surrounding sidewalk pavement
	g. Lower lockers in bath houses reserved for persons in wheel chairs
2. Telephone	2. a. Open telephone station
	b. 32 inches clear entrance
	c. Relatively low dial, receiver, and coin drop
	d. Push button telephones
	e. Adjustable audio control device to increase volume
3. Pier fishing: traditional fishing pier	3. a. Wide access walk to pier
	b. Handrail around entire pier
	c. Arm and pole rests
	d. Kick plate around edges of pier (preventing wheelchairs from going off pier)
	e. Nonslip access walk and pier surface

continued

Table 4. (*Continued*)

Standard facility	Modified facility
4. Vending machine	4. a. Placed in accessible area (for wheelchair access) b. Familiar item logos conspicuously present on the machine (actual items should be in view) c. Easy grip handles or push button operation d. Item indicators well lit
5. Public swimming beach	5. a. Concrete access walk leading from bath house into water b. 32-inch high handrail accompanying walk c. Swimming area not less than 30 square feet and not exceeding depth of 3 feet for the nonswimmer
6. Playground equipment: slides swings sandbox	6. a. Avoid rough surfaces around play area b. Enclosed area with fences to avoid losing balls and equipment c. Play areas must be level and provide adequate space to prevent collisions d. No ladders or legs—gently sloping walk-up ramps e. Grab bars along ramps and on tops and bottoms of slides f. Box-type swings g. Mounded sandboxes with recessed areas to accommodate child in wheelchair
7. Water fountain	7. a. Sprouts and controls located in front of fountain b. Hand and foot operated controls c. Not more than 34 inches from ground d. If fountain higher than 36 inches is used, additional fountain no higher than 30 inches must be adjacent e. Room corners cannot be used for fountain locations

or hobby. The sole purpose of a leadup activity is to prepare the individual for full participation in the original activity. Often several leadup activities may be chained together to teach specific skills necessary for successful engagement in a recreational pursuit. For example, a player can learn many of the skills involved in volleyball by participating in the game of newcomb. The concepts of returning the ball over the net, scoring team points, and the rotation of players can all be learned during newcomb activity. However, since newcomb only requires the participant to catch and throw the ball over the net, an additional leadup activity may have to be implemented to develop the skills necessary for tapping the ball over the net. This can be accomplished by having the players form a circle while taking turns tapping the ball to the player in the circle's center. Thus, by learning more complex activity in small steps, full participation can eventually be facilitated. Nevertheless, a severely physically handicapped individual may never be capable of mastering all the component skills necessary for engagement in the original activity. In this case, the leadup activity may come to serve as a rewarding recreational experience in itself. A person who cannot roller or ice skate, skills necessary for participation in roller or ice hockey, may still be able to play floor hockey successfully, certainly a legitimate sport in its own right.

A number of leadup activities have been developed that can aid in preparation for participation in a baseball game. Among some of the more original are the games of one base, whiffle ball, and fongo baseball. An adjustable batting tee is available that can act as a tool for modified play or as a leadup to hitting a pitched ball, a significantly more difficult skill (Thomas, 1974; Wehman & Schleien, 1979). The tee is economically practical as it can be raised from 27 to 43 inches depending on the height of the batter and can be used with any size ball. Additionally, a ball can be attached to a rope and suspended from the ceiling. This technique allows the batter to practice his swing while eliminating the continuous retrieval of baseballs. See Table 5 for additional examples of leadup activity adaptations.

The five types of adaptations described above represent the primary ways in which a creative teacher or therapist can reduce failure and

Table 5. Leadup activity adaptations for leisure skills

Standard skill	Easier/modified activities
1. Speaking on telephone	1. a. Practice telephone conversation skills using tape recorder
	b. Practice pay phone skills using cardboard mockup and pokerchip currency
2. Baseball	2. a. Kickball to learn concepts of scoring runs, running bases, fielding, etc.
	b. Punchball to develop gross motor coordination
	c. Tee ball to practice batting swing and hitting any size ball
	d. Suspend ball from ceiling for continuous batting practice
	e. Whiffle ball: slower, safer version of baseball

continued

Table 5. (*Continued*)

Standard skill	Easier/modified activities
3. Basketball	3. a. Lay-up line for shooting practice b. Dribbling relays c. "Game of 21" for gaining competition concepts and shooting practice
4. Tennis	4. Rebound practice against wall to practice forehand and backhand strokes
5. Needlework	5. a. Use of lacing board with plastic needle attached to nylon cord b. Sewing block (large plastic box with holes) allowing large plastic needle with rope attached to pass through c. Sewing cards to learn basic movements necessary for sewing and embroidery
6. Cycling	6. a. Training wheels to stabilize bicycle b. Large adult tricycle to minimize balance problems associated with two-wheelers c. Exercise bicycle to practice peddling and increase leg strength and cardiovascular endurance
7. Darts: totaling points	7. a. Cricket requiring player to count number of darts thrown on board instead of adding numbers b. Using numbers 1 through 6 as designated scoring numbers rather than 15 through 20 as usually done in Cricket, allowing for easier number identification

frustration for severely handicapped persons. Although it is imperative that these adaptations be individualized (i.e., not provided for the group as a whole), and temporary, in as many situations as possible, it is certain that without the above described modifications, recreational involvement by many severely handicapped individuals will be nonexistent or minimal at best.

Leisure Skills Curricula Using Adaptations

Leisure skills and adapted physical education curricula have addressed the use of material and procedural adaptations, activity guidelines, and leadup skills to enhance recreational participation. The three curricula presented below have adapted literally hundreds of recreational and physical activities.

The *I Can Curriculum*, developed by the Field Service Unit for Physical Education and Recreation for the Handicapped at Michigan State University in 1976, under the direction of Dr. Janet Wessel, recommends and describes leadup activities and other games that can be played to teach specific game skills. The acquisition of these skills, in turn, enhances successful participation in the more popular activities. The physical education curriculum is divided into four content areas including fundamental skills, aquatics, body management, and health/fitness.

Bender and Valletutti (1976) in their *Leisure Time Skills Curriculum* for the moderately and severely handicapped asked parents and teachers to encourage the handicapped student to seek a variety of interesting leisure time activities. They discouraged the nonproductive skills such as watching television without regard to programming. In order to engage in leisure time activities in a manner that allows him to function as optimally as possible, Bender and Valletutti listed a number of activity guidelines and rule modifications that can be implemented to enhance participation in a specified leisure skill. For instance, an individual who is unable to grasp the rules of the card game, solitaire, can be taught to play a simplified version. The player can learn to shuffle the cards and put them into piles in accordance with their respective color, suit, or number. The game can thus be modified to meet the functioning level of each player.

Because of the various physical, social, and intellectual limitations of developmentally disabled persons, Wehman and Schleien (1979) believed it is essential at times to design and modify recreational activities to meet their special needs. With the assistance of physical, occupational, and recreational therapists, the authors attempted to simplify over 600 activities within their *Leisure Skills Curriculum for Developmentally Disabled Persons*. They included adapted materials, altered environments, and identified leadup skills to permit the severely handicapped to participate. It was stressed that teachers and therapists need to be creative and innovative during the program planning and curriculum implementation process. Wehman and Schleien believe almost all the objects, games, hobbies, and sports played by nonhandicapped individuals can also be enjoyed by the most limited persons. For example, tennis can be carried out with more easily controlled smaller and lighter rackets, enlarged handles, a lower net, smaller court dimensions, and by increasing the number of players per team. The desirability of improving readiness skills of participants through leadup activities, in which they could learn the fundamentals of holding the racket, serving, and hitting forehand before actually competing in a tennis match, was also discussed.

SUMMARY AND RECOMMENDATIONS

A leisure skill adaptation can be a valuable and necessary programming tool. Many times a severely handicapped individual will require a modified or simplified version of an activity in order to participate, succeed, and enjoy. Without such adaptations, recreational pursuits, for many would be impossible and numerous opportunities for rewarding, constructive, and creative experiences unattainable. Therefore, this chapter was designed to facilitate the use of leisure skills adaptations to meet this end. The rationale, historical background, and philosophies of modifying recreational activities were reviewed.

Five types of adaptations were described including material, procedural/rule, skill sequence, community-based facility, and leadup activity. Suggested guidelines to consider when implementing adaptations were also addressed answering questions of the what, when, and how of modified programming. Because minimal research is available concerning the effectiveness and application of skill modifications in various recreational settings, the authors make the following recommendations for further research to overcome the weaknesses in this critical programming area.

Empirical studies investigating the effectiveness and feasibility of adapting recreational activities

Studies comparing and contrasting various activity modifications and implementation methods

Research exploring the effects of adapting activities on mainstreaming and normalization

An examination of the cost effectiveness and feasibility of using adapted materials and equipment as compared to the many hours spent training individuals to use standardized equipment

An examination of the cost effectiveness and feasibility of using homemade or teacher-made versus commercially purchased materials and equipment

Greater attention directed toward the development of community-based facility adaptations to meet the criteria of recent state and federal legislation

As an aid to recreation and educational professionals programming in the leisure area, curricula utilizing the various types of adaptations are reviewed near the end of the chapter. These resource tools, as well as systematically designed published studies and compilation source books, are valuable assets to all workers in the field.

REFERENCES

Adams, R. Putt-putt golf. *Journal of Health, Physical Education and Recreation*, 42(2), 1971.

Adams, R., Daniel, A., & Rullman, L. *Games, sports and exercises for the physically handicapped.* Philadelphia: Lea and Febiger, 1975.

Allen, R. Experiments with bowling. *Best of Challenge, I,* September, 1967.

Amary, I. *Creative recreation for the mentally retarded.* Springfield, IL: Charles C Thomas, 1975.

American Alliance for Health, Physical Education and Recreation. *Making physical education and recreation facilities accessible to all . . . planning . . . designing . . . adapting.* Washington, DC: AAHPER/IRUC, May, 1977.

American Alliance for Health, Physical Education and Recreation. Adapted equipment for physical activities. *Practical Pointers, 1*(5), October, 1977.

Bender, M., & Valletutti, P. *Teaching the moderately and severely handicapped: Curriculum objectives, strategies and activities.* Baltimore: University Park Press, 1976.

Bolt, Martha. Softball for the blind student. *Journal of Health, Physical Education and Recreation, 41*(3), 1970.

Brannan, S. (Ed.). *Our new challenge: Recreation for the deaf-blind.* Seattle: Northwest Regional Center for Deaf-Blind Children, Community Services Division, Department of Social and Health Services, July, 1975.

Brown, L., Branston-McClean, M., Baumgart, D., Vincent, L., Falvey, M., & Schroeder, J. Using the characteristics of current and subsequent least restrictive environments in the development of curricular content for severely handicapped students. *AAESPH Review, 4*(4), 1979.

Carlson, B., & Ginglend, D. *Recreation for retarded teenagers and young adults.* Nashville: Abingdon Press, 1968.

Cowart, J. *Instructional aids for adaptive physical education.* Hayward, CA: Alameda County School Department, 1973 (ERIC Document Reproduction Service No. ED 106 341).

Detwiler, B., Merrill, D., & Robinson, J. Summertime fun. *The Exceptional Parent, 5*(3), 1975.

Earle, P. & Yost, G. Sports, athletics and games for the deaf-blind. In S. Brannon (Ed.), *Our new challenge: Recreation for the deaf-blind.* Seattle: Northwest Regional Center for Deaf-Blind Children, Community Services Division, Department of Social and Health Services, July, 1975.

Easter Seal Society of Massachusetts. Wheel about garden. *The Exceptional Parent, 5*(3), 1975.

Florida Learning Resources System. *Teacher-made materials.* Ocala, FL: Florida Learning Resources System, 1976. (ERIC Document Reproduction Service No. ED 133 971).

Ford, J., & Duckworth, B. *Physical management for the quadriplegic patient.* Philadelphia: F. A. Davis Company, 1976.

Geddes, D. *Physical activities for individuals with handicapping conditions.* St. Louis: C. V. Mosby Company, 1978.

Geddes, D., & Burnette, W. *Physical education and recreation for impaired, disabled and handicapped individuals . . . past, present and future.* Washington, DC: Information and Research Utilization Center, 1975. (ERIC Document Reproduction Service No. ED 119 396).

Goldsmith, S. *Designing for the disabled: A manual of technical information.* London: RIBA Technical Information Service, 1963.

Grosse, S. Indoor target golf. *Journal of Health, Physical Education and Recreation, 42*(1), 1971.

Gunn, S., & Peterson, C. *Therapeutic recreation program design: Principles and procedures.* Englewood Cliffs, NJ: Prentice-Hall, Inc., 1978.

Hunt, V. *Recreation for the handicapped.* Englewood Cliffs, NJ: Prentice-Hall, Inc., 1955.

Information and Research Utilization Center. *Physical activities for impaired, disabled and handicapped individuals.* Washington, DC: IRUC, 1976.

Kraus, R. *Therapeutic recreation service: Principles and practices.* Philadelphia: W. B. Saunders Company, 1973.

Lear, R. *Play helps: Toys and activities for handicapped children.* London: William Heinemann Medical Books Ltd., 1977.

Lewis, J. *Mock baseball and scrub.* Vancouver, B.C., Canada: Canadian National Institute for the Blind, 1970.

Mason, R. *Bowling for the handicapped.* Washington, DC: American Alliance for Health, Physical Education and Recreation, Programs for the Handicapped, May 1969.

Nesbitt, J., Brown, P., & Murphy, J. *Recreation and leisure service for the disadvantaged.* Philadelphia: Lea and Febiger, 1970.

O'Morrow, G. *Therapeutic recreation: A helping profession.* Reston, VA: Reston Publishing Company, 1976.

Pomeroy, J. *Recreation for the physically handicapped.* New York: Macmillan Company, 1964.

Ries, M. *Design standards to accommodate people with physical disabilities in parks and open space planning.* Unpublished Dissertation, Graduate School of Landscape Architecture, University of Wisconsin, Madison, 1973.

Robinault, I. (Ed.). *Functional aids for the multiply handicapped.* New York: Harper and Row, 1973.

Schleichkorn, J., & Sirianni, F. Tournament bowling: An activity for the handicapped. *Journal of Health, Physical Education and Recreation, 43*(9), 1972.

Schleien, S., & Kiernan, J. Leisure skills programming for severely/profoundly handicapped persons. *Virginia Views* (VRPS), *1*(1), 1980.

Sherman, H. Hands on hobbies. In S. Brannon (Ed.) *Our new challenge: Recreation for the deaf-blind.* Seattle: Northwest Regional Center for Deaf-Blind Children, Community Services Division, Department of Social and Health Services, July, 1975.

Thomas, W. *A physical education program for adults and young adults; Designed for use with moderately, severely and profoundly mentally retarded.* South Bend, IN: Council for the Retarded of Saint Joseph County, Inc., IRUC, 1974.

Tillman, A. *The program book for recreation professionals.* Palo Alto, CA: National Press Books, 1973.

Virginia Commission of Outdoor Recreation—Recreation Services Section. *Architectural accessibility for the disabled in park and recreation facilities.* Richmond: Virginia Commission of Outdoor Recreation, 1976.

Wehman, P. *Helping the mentally retarded acquire play skills: A behavioral approach.* Springfield, IL: Charles C Thomas, 1977.

Wehman, P., & Schleien, S. *Leisure skills curriculum for developmentally disabled persons.* Richmond, VA: School of Education, Virginia Commonwealth University, 1979.

Wessel, J. *I can physical education program.* Northbrook, IL: Hubbard Scientific Co., 1976.

Wolfensberger, W. *The principle of normalization in human services.* Toronto, Canada: National Institute on Mental Retardation, 1972.

Chapter 5
CURRICULUM DESIGN AND FORMAT

The purpose of this chapter is to describe the format of the leisure curriculum that follows in the next four chapters. As is evident in Table 1, an effort has been made to develop a uniform program format that corresponds to the necessary components of an individualized education program (IEP) or an individualized habilitation plan (IHP).

The format of the curriculum includes:

1. A program goal
2. An instructional objective (short-term)
3. A task analysis of each skill
4. The verbal cue required for instruction in the skill
5. Materials that are required for instruction
6. Teaching procedures and special adaptations with each skill

These program components comprise a systematic approach to leisure instruction and have been detailed in Chapter 4.

ACTIVITY GROUPINGS: DESCRIPTION AND RATIONALE

It was a difficult task to pinpoint a minimum number of serviceable activity categories that would encompass all the recreation/leisure skills that were generated. The four activity categories that were decided upon (object manipulation, games, hobbies, sports), however, encompass many skills within the leisure skill area. It is expected that teachers, recreation therapists, or parents should easily be able to locate activities appropriate for handicapped individuals.

The four major activity headings are not intended to bind the instructor, but, on the contrary, to give the teacher/leader leeway to utilize several kinds of leisure skills that fall into the different activity areas. While continuity is vital, we encourage teaching participants skills from each of the categories, assuming that the skills presented are appropriate for the individual's age group and present ability levels. Among the four categories, over 600 activities were initially identified. In this text only a relatively small proportion are presented. The four activity groups are listed below with descriptions for each.

Table 1. Program format

Name of Activity:

Instructional Objective:
Materials:
Verbal Cue:

Task Analysis:

Activity Guidelines/Special Adaptations:

Object Manipulation (Toy Play)

Leisure skills falling into this activity group are the most basic form of recreation/leisure participation outside of self-stimulation. They involve interaction with an inanimate object by the participant. The object is the focus of the individual's attention and is not usually part of a larger game.

Usually no rules exist during object manipulation or toy play activity, and therefore, the individual may design his own activity for use with the object. Objects are selected to stimulate solitary activity and to allow the individual to express himself and exercise acquired abilities in each phase of development. *The most practical objects tend to be those that have the widest range of possible application.*

Games

Games are recreational activities that involve definite rules ranging from simple to high functioning level for participation. They may or may not involve the manipulation of objects or toys. A game can involve competition and/or cooperation of participants and usually involves more than one person. The participants must learn to take turns and abide by the rules. An intended outcome must be inherent in the game. As in the sports category, the concept of winning and losing is introduced. However, games are the purest form of recreation in that they are played because the participants enjoy playing that particular game. Sheer pleasure is the primary motivating factor. This activity category includes board and table games, social (get acquainted) games, gross motor games, musical/rhythmical games, and card games.

Hobbies

Hobbies are recreational activities that have potential to become lifelong leisure skills. An individual may pursue a hobby as a youngster and continue to excel in and utilize those skills with increasing degrees of sophistication throughout his or her lifetime. Participation in hobbies tends to be less active than in either sports or other physical games.

Curriculum Design and Format 91

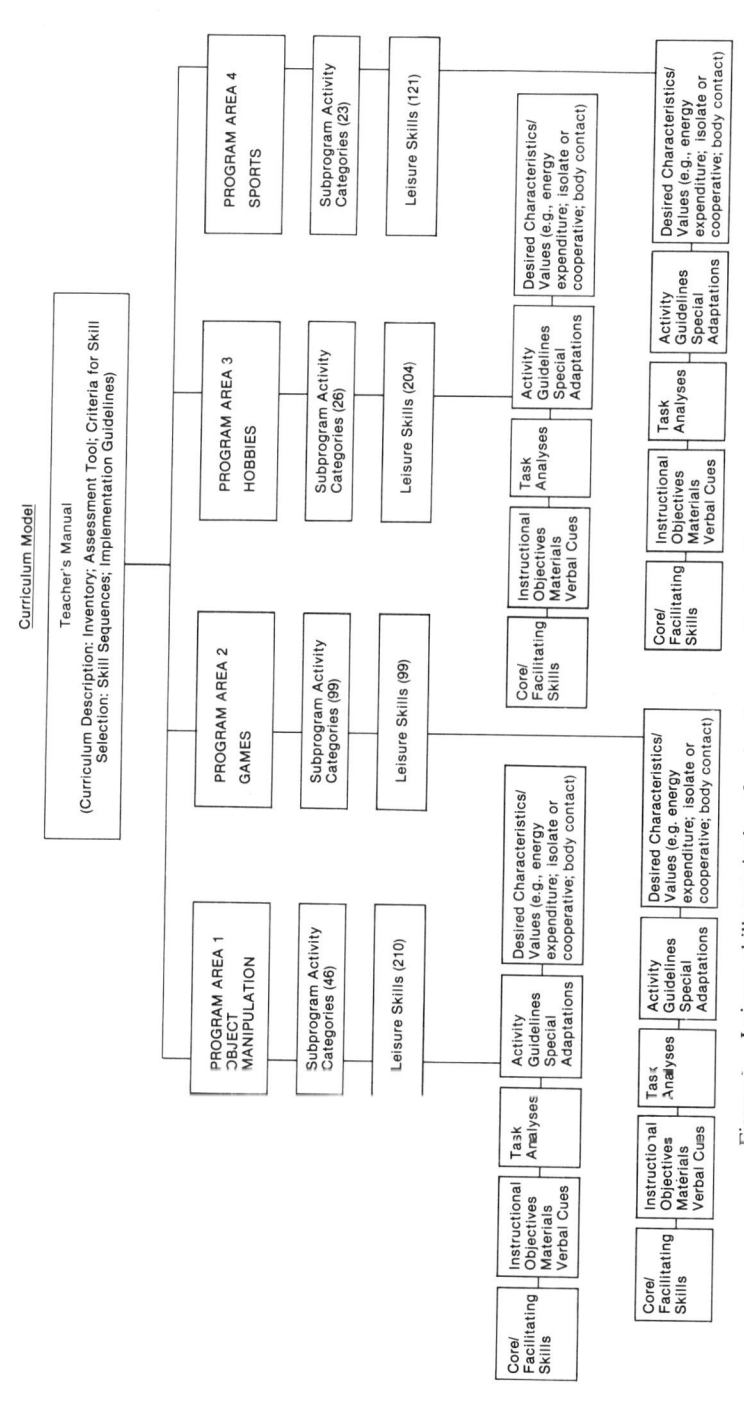

Figure 1. Leisure skills curriculum for developmentally disabled persons: Virginia model (LSCDD).

Hobbies may include activities such as stamp and coin collecting, playing a musical instrument, and a wide variety of arts and crafts activities. A hobby is usually a solitary pursuit, and therefore, noncompetitive; the concepts of "win and lose" do not exist. While it is hoped that an interest in many of the different leisure skills would continuously develop throughout a person's lifetime, it is typically the skills in the hobby activity category that are most enduring for the individual.

Sports

The distinction between sports and games is often characterized by a time line. Although activities falling in both categories employ a definite set of rules, the rules and equipment used in sports tend to be more sophisticated. With sports there also tends to be a greater emphasis placed on the competitive aspects of the activity. Both individual and team sports are incorporated into the curriculum requiring various degrees of social and motor coordination ability levels. Disabled persons are becoming more active in sports nationwide, as can be observed by the increased interest in Special Olympics and wheelchair sports and games for both children and adults.

In reviewing many leisure skills and recreation materials, most activities seemed to cluster predominantly around one of these four activity groups. Clearly, a skill might belong in more than one category, but for ease of organization, we have placed it in the category considered to be most appropriate. Figure 1 depicts the overall curriculum design.

SKILL SEQUENCING

Six hundred leisure skills were identified and field-tested in the four program areas. A review of the four chapters reveals that not all of the skills have been included. We have not attempted to sequence skills within each curriculum chapter for two reasons. First, designing a leisure skills program should not necessarily be implementing a motor skill program. For this reason, it was felt that simply sequencing all skills developmentally would be inconsistent with the purpose of developing a *repertoire* of leisure skills. Second, there is tremendous difficulty in taking all leisure skills and sequencing them developmentally. Many recreational activities do not align themselves developmentally as easily as language and basic motor skills.

Our solution to these problems has been to:

1. provide a developmental/logical sequence of motor actions that are in each program volume; this will help select skills appropriate for an individual's level of functioning, and
2. provide core skills for each chapter that will help a teacher decide

what the basic motor and cognitive skills are for performing the given activities.

CORE SKILLS

Core skills are basic motor and cognitive skills that facilitate participation in the leisure skills program. Although the curriculum's activities can be specially adapted to meet the relative abilities of most participants, the appropriate leisure skills can effectively be utilized to teach the core skills within the context of the activity. The core skills are not prerequisite skills that are necessary for the individual to participate in a leisure activity. It should be noted that in addition to implementing leisure activities, the core skills are also essential for the acquisition of many functional self-help and everyday community living skills. The motor and cognitive skills below have been identified as the components linked with the development of leisure skills and human growth. The core skills are:

1. *Head Control.* The ability to hold the head erect. The ability to maintain the head position at the midline of the body is necessary for all movements as well as sitting and standing independently. This skill is typically acquired at 2 months of age.
2. *Attending/Focusing.* When head control is acquired, the person has potential to utilize mental concentration or readiness to commence an activity. It is this ability to focus and concentrate on a specified stimulus, whether it be a person's voice, musical sound, physical action, or object, in order to respond appropriately to that stimulus. Without the ability to attend, the participant will be unable to initiate a desired response.
3. *Visual/Auditory Tracking.* A cognitive/motor skill that involves the movement of the head (head turn) or eyes (scanning) to follow the path of an object or sound. The individual's ability to move about and to act upon the environment is dependent upon locating and avoiding objects around him. Visual tracking is normally acquired at approximately 5 months of age.
4. *Object Permanence.* The ability to search for an object that is temporarily out of the individual's sight. With the acquisition of this skill, the object will continue to exist even though it is not in sight. Initially, this limited cognitive ability is present until the individual is able to visually track an object. When this concept has been grasped, the participant will attempt to search for an object that is not in sight, such as a tennis ball that has been hit out of bounds or a golf ball that has been hit into a hole and is temporarily out of view.
5. *Means/Ends.* A cognitive skill that allows the individual to use an

appropriate means to reach a goal and obtain a result. Upon acquisition of this skill, the participant understands that in order to watch a television program (end), a knob (means) must be manipulated. Spinning a dial in order to move a playing piece during a game requires this same understanding. This knowledge allows for the generalization of a skill to a variety of situations.

6. *Palmar Grasp.* A fine motor skill that involves the wrapping of the fingers and thumb of a hand around an object to control the movement of that object, such as the handle of a frying pan, a tennis racket, or a drinking glass.

7. *Pincer Grasp.* A fine motor skill involving the thumb and index finger. These two fingers are brought together on either side of an object to control the movement of that object. This grasp is generally used to manipulate fairly small and/or lightweight objects such as a sheet of paper, or a piece of candy, or used to pick up a pencil. The individual normally acquires this skill at age 12 months.

8. *Arm/Leg Extension (Reaching, Pushing).* The ability to straighten the arm or leg away from midline when initially in a bent position. Arm extension is used in several skills such as throwing, reaching, and pushing. Leg extension is necessary for walking, running, and kicking.

9. *Arm/Leg Flexion (Pulling).* Involves bending of the arm or leg toward midline usually in conjunction with limb extension. Arm and leg flexion are used in many of the same skills as arm and leg extension.

10. *Controlled Hand Release.* Involves the participant's loosening of a pincer or palmar grasp, or any other in order to let go of an object. Any skill that requires grasping an object will additionally require the participant's voluntary release of that object. Typically, an object may be released by opening the hand to expose the palm and extending the fingers.

11. *Sitting Unsupported.* Involves holding the upper trunk erect while resting the lower trunk on a chair or the floor. It may be the most appropriate position for a nonambulatory person to engage in a leisure skill. In the absence of this skill, the participant can utilize braces to give support while seated, or sit in a wheelchair. Sitting independently normally occurs at age 9 months.

12. *Standing Unsupported.* Involves holding the upper and lower trunk erect with both feet positioned on the floor. This skill is necessary for participation in most sports and motor games. However, if this skill is not acquired, many activities can be adapted to a seated position. A device can be purchased or constructed that will support the individual in an erect position (Hammett Co.). Standing unsupported normally occurs at age 12 months.

FIELD TESTING

The field testing process was incorporated into the curriculum's development to verify the 600 task analyses. Teachers at local public schools serving severely multiply handicapped students in Virginia responded to questions such as: Are all the steps required to perform the skill present in the task analysis?; Is there a logical progression of steps?; Is the task analysis coherent? Other inquiries concerning instructional objectives, verbal cues, special materials and/or environmental adaptations, and overall impressions regarding the organization and practical aspects of the leisure skills were considered. Below are the guidelines used in field testing.

Do the steps in the task analysis follow a logical sequence?
Are the steps in the task analysis coherent?
Is the skill broken down into small enough and a sufficient number of steps to be relevant to the abilities of developmentally disabled persons of all ability levels?
Are there any steps missing from the task analysis? If so, what steps need to be added?
Have the activity guidelines/special adaptations been advantageous to you when teaching the skill?
Are there any activity guidelines or special adaptations, not already mentioned, that are worth adding to the program form in order to make the skill relevant to the abilities of even the most profoundly disabled individual?
Is the instructional objective clearly stated?
Does the instructional objective state specifically what needs to be accomplished by the participant?
Is the verbal cue appropriate and clearly stated?
What are your overall impressions and suggestions regarding the organization and practical aspects of the skill?

Chapter 6
HOBBIES

Hobbies are activities that are performed after work hours by persons of all ages. They are long-term leisure pursuits that an individual may participate in throughout an entire lifetime. In order to pursue a hobby, one must initially have an opportunity and/or interest in the activities or skills involved, have access to the materials/equipment needed, if any, and acquire the necessary techniques. A hobby's lifelong nature allows an individual to continuously acquire new skills and knowledge. Hobbies are considered true leisure activities because the goal of hobby participation is to derive pleasure, whether it is by creating, collecting, listening, observing, or learning.

The hobby skills in this chapter include:

Age Level*	Hobby Skills	Page
	BOOKS AND MAGAZINES	
C/A	Turn Pages in Magazine	98
C/A	Find Seat in Library	99
	CAMPING	
C/A	Roast Marshmallows	100
C/A	Use of Sleeping Bag	101
	COOKING	
C/A	Make Kool-Aid	102
C/A	Make Peanut Butter and Jelly Sandwich	103
	CYCLING	
C/A	Peddle Cycle	104
C/A	Balance and Steer Cycle	105
	HOLIDAY ACTIVITY	
C/A	Decorate Christmas Tree	106
C	Decorate Easter Egg	107
	MUSICAL/RHYTHMICAL INSTRUMENTS	
C/A	Shake Maraca (rattle) to Beat	108
C/A	Play Tambourine	109
	PET CARE	
C/A	Walk Dog On Leash	110
C/A	Feed Dog	111
C/A	Use of Pooper-Scooper	112
	PHOTOGRAPHY	
C/A	Use of Instamatic Camera	113
C/A	Make Photograph Album	115

* C, Indicates chronologically age-appropriate for child; A, Indicates chronologically age-appropriate for adolescent and adult; C/A, Indicates chronologically age-appropriate for child, adolescent, and adult.

	PLANT CARE	
C/A	Plant Seed	116
C/A	Water and Mist Plant	117
	SPECTATOR LEISURE/COMMUNITY EVENTS	
C/A	Go To Movie Theater	118
C/A	Attend Social Dance	118
	SPECTATOR LEISURE/HOME	
C/A	Use of Record Player	119
C/A	Use of Television	121
	SUNBATHING	
C/A	Put On Bathing Suit	121
C/A	Put on Suntan Lotion	122
	TABLE GAME HOBBIES	
C/A	Play Foosball	123
C/A	Play Pinball	124
C/A	Play Electric Bowling	125
C/A	Play Pool	126

BOOKS AND MAGAZINES

Name of Activity: Turn Pages in Magazine

Instructional Objective: Given a magazine on a shelf, the participant will remove the book from the shelf and turn through 5 pages, one at a time, allowing 4 seconds between page turns, 80% of the time.
Materials: magazine, shelf
Verbal Cue: "Patti, look through the magazine."

Task Analysis:
1. Walk to book shelf.
2. Extend dominant hand with fingers extended toward magazine.
3. Grasp opposite sides of magazine with dominant hand using pincer grasp.
4. Take magazine off shelf by bending at elbow.
5. Grasp bottom right hand corner of cover with nondominant hand using pincer grasp.
6. Open magazine by moving hand in semicircular arc, turning first page.
7. Look at open page of magazine for at least 4 seconds.
8. Turn second page and look at it for at least 4 seconds.
9. Turn third page.
10. Turn fourth page.
11. Turn fifth page.

Activity Guidelines/Special Adaptations:
1. The magazine can be placed flat on the shelf so participant with poor muscular or fine motor control may slide book from shelf.
2. Participant may use two hands to remove book from shelf.
3. For participants having difficulty with fine motor control, the bottom right-hand corners of the magazine can be reinforced with thin cardboard. Clothespins could also be attached to the pages and used to turn them.
4. A small colorful magazine can be made from construction paper that may make it easier for participant to grasp and turn the pages.
5. If there is a problem with the magazine sliding around the desk or table, the magazine can be secured to the table by running a string across the inside spine of the magazine between the two center pages and then tying it around the table.

Name of Activity: Find Seat in Library

Instructional Objective: Upon entering the library, the participant will find a seat at a vacant table, 80% of the time.
Materials: library, chair
Verbal Cue: "Patti, find a seat."

Task Analysis:
1. Enter library.
2. Walk to area where tables and chairs are located.
3. Walk to a vacant table.
4. Stand directly behind and to the side of chair.
5. Grasp back of chair with dominant hand using palmar grasp.
6. Pull chair out away from table by moving hand backward toward body.
7. Stand directly in front of chair, facing table.
8. Bend at both knees, lowering body to chair seat, and assume sitting position.
9. Grasp sides of seat with both hands using palmar grasp.
10. Lean forward slightly by bending forward at waist.
11. Pull chair forward by moving hands toward table until abdomen is 8 inches from edge of table.

Activity Guidelines/Special Adaptations:
1. This activity can be simulated in classroom as a leadup activity. Several chairs and tables can be set up, with participants seated randomly. Have participant enter room and locate seat at vacant table.

2. It is important to stress to participants that privacy of people in the library should be respected. If there is not a vacant seat, participant should sit as far away as possible from another person at a table, so as not to disturb reading and studying of others.
3. Nonambulatory participants need to find wide enough space at table to accommodate wheelchair.

CAMPING

Name of Activity: Roast Marshmallows

Instructional Objective: Given a campfire, a marshmallow, and a stick at least 3 feet long, the participant will roast a marshmallow, 80% of the time.
Materials: campfire, marshmallow, stick (at least 3 feet long)
Verbal Cue: "Janet, roast the marshmallow."

Task Analysis:
1. Grasp narrow end of stick with dominant hand using palmar grasp.
2. Grasp marshmallow with nondominant hand using pincer grasp.
3. Position end of stick directly in front of marshmallow.
4. Push end of stick completely through center of marshmallow by moving stick toward marshmallow.
5. Release marshmallow onto stick by extending fingers of nondominant hand.
6. Grasp end of stick opposite marshmallow with dominant hand using palmar grasp.
7. Stand 2 feet away from campfire.
8. Position marshmallow directly above flames by extending arm at elbow.
9. Hold marshmallow over flames, turning it periodically, until all sides of marshmallow turn slightly brown.

Activity Guidelines/Special Adaptations:
1. This activity may be practiced by holding a marshmallow over a candle in the classroom.
2. It may be helpful to sharpen the end of the stick to allow marshmallow to be put on the stick more easily.
3. Metal clothes hangers are sometimes used rather than sticks to eliminate the possibility of the stick catching on fire. Also, a wire handle can be constructed to provide ease in holding the stick. However, since the metal conducts heat, participants may wish to wear a glove or use a rag to hold the hanger while roasting.

4. The marshmallow will best be roasted by holding the marshmallow *above* the flames rather than *in* the flames to avoid burning it. Marshmallow should be allowed to cool before eating it.

Name of Activity: Use of Sleeping Bag

Instructional Objective: Given a sleeping bag, the participant will unroll, unzip, and lie in the sleeping bag, 80% of the time.
Materials: sleeping bag
Verbal Cue: "Janet, lie in the sleeping bag."

Task Analysis:
1. Grasp 2 loose ends of knot on sleeping bag with both hands using pincer grasp.
2. Untie knot by moving hands away from each other.
3. Place palms of both hands on top of rolled up sleeping bag.
4. Unroll bag completely by extending arms at elbows and walking forward.
5. Grasp head of zipper on side of sleeping bag with dominant hand using pincer grasp.
6. Unzip bag by extending arm at elbow.
7. Release zipper by extending fingers.
8. Grasp top layer of sleeping bag with dominant hand using palmar grasp.
9. Expose inside of sleeping bag by lifting top layer up and away from zippered side of bag.
10. Sit inside sleeping bag.
11. Grasp head of zipper inside bag with dominant hand using pincer grasp.
12. Zip bag up by bending arm at elbow.
13. Lie in sleeping bag.

Activity Guidelines/Special Adaptations:
1. To simplify this activity, the sleeping bag can be unrolled and unzipped before participant begins activity.
2. The head of the zipper may be enlarged by wrapping it with adhesive tape to make grasping and zipping easier.
3. To foster social cooperation, participants can help each other zip up their sleeping bags. The teacher can zip up the remaining participant's bag.
4. It should be stressed that the campfire be extinguished before campers go to sleep. Teach participants the fire prevention slogan of Smokey the Bear who says, "Only you can prevent forest fires."

COOKING

Name of Activity: Make Kool-Aid

Instructional Objective: Given a package of Kool-Aid, ½-gallon water pitcher, long-handled spoon, and water faucet, the participant will make a pitcher of Kool-Aid, 80% of the time.

Materials: package of Kool-Aid, ½-gallon water pitcher, long-handled spoon, water faucet

Verbal Cue: "Art, make a pitcher of Kool-Aid."

Task Analysis:
1. Grasp opposite sides of opened package of Kool-Aid with dominant hand using palmar grasp.
2. Raise package to level parallel with rim of pitcher by bending at elbow.
3. Empty contents of package into pitcher by rotating wrist downward, simultaneously moving open end of package toward center of pitcher.
4. Place empty package on table by lowering hand to table and extending fingers.
5. Grasp handle of pitcher with dominant hand using palmar grasp.
6. Lift pitcher off table by bending at elbow.
7. Carry pitcher to water faucet.
8. Position pitcher directly below water faucet.
9. Grasp cold water knob with dominant hand using palmar grasp.
10. Turn cold water on by rotating wrist in appropriate direction.
11. Fill pitcher to water level marked on pitcher.
12. Turn cold water off by rotating wrist in appropriate direction.
13. Carry pitcher back to table.
14. Release grasp on pitcher by extending fingers.
15. Grasp spoon with dominant hand using palmar grasp.
16. Position bowl of spoon directly above center of pitcher.
17. Lower spoon into pitcher by lowering arm at shoulder.
18. Rotate wrist in a circular motion to mix Kool-Aid and water.
19. Continue using spoon to thoroughly mix Kool-Aid and water (until Kool-Aid is completely dissolved in water).

Activity Guidelines/Special Adaptations:
1. Initially, the package of Kool-Aid can be opened before participant begins this activity. Eventually, participant should be required to open the package on his own.
2. A line should be marked on the pitcher to indicate the correct water level.
3. Kool-Aid also comes in large tin cans that have a pre-measured scoop

inside. This would be more economical and may be easier for some participants to manipulate than a package of Kool-Aid.
4. A long-handled wooden cooking spoon would be appropriate for use in this activity.
5. Plastic pitchers are lighter and easier for participants to carry; also, the danger of breaking a glass container is eliminated.

Name of Activity: Make Peanut Butter and Jelly Sandwich

Instructional Objective: Given a jar of peanut butter, a jar of jelly, a table knife, and 2 slices of bread, the participant will prepare a peanut butter and jelly sandwich, 80% of the time.
Materials: jar of peanut butter, jar of jelly, table knife, 2 slices of bread
Verbal Cue: "Art, make a peanut butter and jelly sandwich."

Task Analysis:
1. Grasp jar of peanut butter with nondominant hand using palmar grasp.
2. Grasp lid of jar with dominant hand using palmar grasp.
3. Turn lid in counterclockwise direction to open jar by rotating wrist.
4. Place lid on table top by lowering hand to table and extending fingers.
5. Release grasp on jar of peanut butter by extending fingers.
6. Open jar of jelly.
7. Spread peanut butter on one slice of bread.
8. Spread jelly on other slice of bread.
9. Grasp adjacent top corners of jellied bread slice with both hands using pincer grasp.
10. Position bottom of jellied slice perpendicular to top of peanut buttered slice with both edges of both slices touching each other.
11. Lower jellied slice onto top of peanut buttered slice by bending at both elbows.
12. Line up both slices of bread to complete peanut butter and jelly sandwich.

Activity Guidelines/Special Adaptations:
1. Although there is no real need to cut the sandwich, the participant or teacher can cut the sandwich in half or quarters to make it easier to eat.
2. The lid of the jar can initially be loosened, making it easier to open.
3. A knife with a wide blade will make it easier to spread ingredients; also, handle of knife can be enlarged or extended.
4. It is easier to spread the ingredients on bread that is a couple of days old and not extremely fresh. There is less chance of the bread tearing as the ingredients are spread on it.

5. Although chunky style peanut butter is preferred by many people, smooth style peanut butter is easier to spread.
6. Cream cheese can be substituted for peanut butter and combined with jelly.

CYCLING

Name of Activity: Peddle Cycle

Instructional Objective: Given a bicycle, the participant will get on the bicycle and peddle it 8 feet without stopping, 80% of the time.
Materials: bicycle
Verbal Cue: "Kathy, get on the bicycle and start peddling."

Task Analysis:
1. Stand on left side of bicycle, facing bicycle seat.
2. Grasp handles with both hands using palmar grasp.
3. Position left foot sideways directly above pedal on left side of bicycle.
4. Place left foot onto pedal, simultaneously shifting body weight to left foot.
5. Raise right leg upward and outward to right side by bending at knee.
6. Bring right leg up and over bicycle seat by extending right leg fully at knee.
7. Lower right foot onto pedal on right side of bicycle.
8. Lower body to bicycle seat by bending at both knees, sitting on bicycle.
9. Place ball of right foot on right pedal.
10. Place ball of left foot on left pedal.
11. Apply downward pressure onto left pedal with left foot by extending left leg at knee, simultaneously bending right leg at knee.
12. Apply downward pressure onto right pedal with right foot by extending at knee, simultaneously bending left leg at knee.
13. Continue alternately bending and extending at knees of both legs simultaneously to peddle cycle 1 foot.
14. Peddle cycle 2 feet.
15. Peddle cycle 3 feet.
16. Peddle cycle 4 feet.
17. Peddle cycle 6 feet.
18. Peddle cycle 8 feet.

Activity Guidelines/Special Adaptations:
1. Although the bicycle can be supported by the kickstand when implementing this activity, it may still be too wobbly for some participants. Training wheels can be attached to the bicycle to stabilize

it. Also, a large adult tricycle can be used instead of a bicycle, minimizing balance problems associated with two-wheelers.
2. An exercise bicycle is immobile and can be used for practice. It is not too difficult to convert a regular bicycle into a stationary one—there are adaptive devices available in most sporting goods stores.
3. The teacher or another participant may hold the bicycle upright to provide stability and support for the participant.
4. Each participant should ride a bicycle or tricycle that matches his or her size. A bicycle that is too large or too small will make cycling a clumsy and dangerous activity.
5. The handgrips of handlebars should have finger indentations or other rough surfaces for increased steering control and to prevent hands from slipping.
6. Participants should wear tight-fitting clothes (no bell bottoms or long, baggy shirt sleeves) when riding the bicycle. By keeping pants and sleeves free from the cycle's chain, danger is significantly reduced. Bicycle safety must be stressed.
7. Even participants who do not have use of their legs can enjoy cycling, since there is a hand-driven tricycle available. The tricycle has a padded leg rest and is powered by turning a left and right crank with the hands. Not only would this provide enjoyment and mobility for the participant, but it would build up the arms and shoulders.
8. In addition to the standard adult tricycle, a more stable 4-wheel tricycle is available. It is specially designed so that pedaling effort is greatly reduced and it has a front and rear basket for carrying.
9. Cycling is an outstanding way to improve breathing, stimulate circulation, increase cardiovascular endurance, improve dynamic balance, and increase muscular strength in arms, legs, back, shoulders, and abdomen. Weight loss is also a positive consequence of bicycling. On the average, a male can burn approximately 500 calories an hour, and a female 300 calories an hour by cycling.
10. There are special adaptive foot support blocks available that shorten the distance to the pedals and have straps to secure the feet in place. These wooden blocks bolt onto the cycle pedals and are available for either children or adults.
11. Since bicycling is a strenuous gross motor activity, it is highly recommended that participants begin with short rides and gradually increase distance.

Name of Activity: Balance and Steer Cycle

Instructional Objective: Given a bicycle, the participant will steer the bicycle using the handlebars without veering from a 10-foot straight line by more than 3 feet on either side, 80% of the time.

Materials: bicycle
Verbal Cue: "Kathy, ride the bicycle."

Task Analysis:
1. Get on bicycle.
2. Propel bicycle forward by peddling the bicycle or by coasting.
3. Steer bicycle along straight course for 1 foot using handlebars.
4. Steer bicycle for 2 feet.
5. Steer bicycle for 4 feet.
6. Steer bicycle for 6 feet.
7. Steer bicycle for 8 feet.
8. Steer bicycle for 10 feet.

Activity Guidelines/Special Adaptations:
1. Training wheels or an adult tricycle can be used if participant has not mastered balancing on the bicycle.
2. Depending on the ability of the participant, the teacher may wish to guide the participant's hands as she steers the bicycle. It is difficult to teach this skill in isolation, apart from peddling and balancing; steering is an integral part of balancing skills when learning to ride a bike.
3. Lines may be drawn on the ground for participant to follow when steering the bicycle. A bright red line can be drawn in the middle and 2 lines drawn on either side of the red line, 3 feet from it. Participant should attempt to steer the bike 10 feet along the red line without crossing over the lines on either side of it.
4. Before any bicyclist attempts to ride a bicycle on a city street, safety precautions should be stressed. These include obeying traffic rules, using reflectors and a headlight for night riding, and wearing brightly colored clothing for easy visibility.
5. Local governments have converted several miles of land into bicycle paths throughout the country. These paths are regulated safety routes for bikers and have been clearly marked to guide the bicyclist and to warn motorists. Participants should be advised to ride on these routes when bicycling outdoors.

HOLIDAY ACTIVITY

Name of Activity: Decorate Christmas Tree

Instructional Objective: Given a Christmas tree and 3 ornaments, the participant will place the ornaments on the tree, 80% of the time.
Materials: Christmas tree, 3 ornaments

Verbal Cue: "Peggy, decorate the Christmas tree."

Task Analysis:
1. Extend dominant hand downward to ornament box, palm faced down.
2. Grasp hook of first ornament with dominant hand using pincer grasp.
3. Raise ornament to branch level by bending arm at elbow.
4. Grasp tree branch with nondominant hand using pincer grasp.
5. Position hook of ornament directly above branch.
6. Hook ornament onto branch by lowering dominant arm at shoulder.
7. Release ornament onto tree branch by extending fingers.
8. Release grasp of branch in nondominant hand by extending fingers.
9. Place second ornament on tree.
10. Place third ornament on tree.

Activity Guidelines/Special Adaptations:
1. Christmas, December 25th, is a holiday celebrating the birth of Jesus Christ. Participants can get involved in several other holiday rituals at this time. Decorating the Christmas tree is just one appropriate leisure time activity that can be performed.
2. Participants can practice placing shower curtain hooks onto dowels or placing clothes hangers on closet rods as a leadup activity. Progress to smaller hooks until participant exhibits proficiency with hooks the same size as those used for Christmas ornaments.
3. Participants can get involved in making their own Christmas ornaments. It would be reinforcing for each participant to be able to hang a personalized ornament on the classroom tree.

Name of Activity: Decorate Easter Egg

Instructional Objective: Given 1 hard boiled egg and coloring dye, the participant will color 1 egg, 80% of the time.
Materials: hard boiled egg, dye kit, cup, spoon, cake cooling rack
Verbal Cue: "Peggy, paint the egg."

Task Analysis:
1. Sit at table in front of egg, spoon, and cups of dye.
2. Grasp spoon with dominant hand using palmar grasp.
3. Grasp egg with nondominant hand using modified pincer grasp.
4. Position egg directly above cradle of spoon.
5. Release egg onto spoon by extending fingers of nondominant hand.
6. Position egg directly above dye cup.
7. Rotate wrist downward to release egg into dye.
8. Allow egg to remain in dye for at least 2 minutes.

9. Position cradle of spoon directly above center of cup.
10. Place cradle of spoon into cup by lowering dominant arm at shoulder, simultaneously rotating wrist downward so that spoon slides under egg.
11. Rotate wrist upward so that it is resting in cradle of spoon.
12. Remove egg from cup by bending at elbow.
13. Position egg directly above cooling rack.
14. Place egg on rack by rotating wrist downward.
15. Wait for egg to dry.

Activity Guidelines/Special Adaptations:
1. Easter is an annual festival in the spring celebrating the resurrection of Jesus Christ. Decorating Easter eggs is just one appropriate leisure time activity that can be performed.
2. Kitchen tongs may be easier than a spoon for the participant when dipping the egg into the dye. Using a large bowl would give the participant a larger target area to aim for when dipping.
3. Although the eggs may be boiled and cooled before giving them to participant to color, the teacher can incorporate the skills involved in boiling the eggs if feasible.
4. Hollow plastic eggs may be substituted for real eggs and used for storing goodies.
5. Younger participants will enjoy preparing for the Easter Bunny and, of course, they will enjoy an Easter egg hunt.

MUSICAL/RHYTHMICAL INSTRUMENTS

Name of Activity: Shake Maraca (Rattle) to Beat

Instructional Objective: Given a maraca and a simple beat, the participant will shake the instrument simultaneously with 3 consecutive beats, 80% of the time.

Materials: maraca (rattle)

Verbal Cue: "Ralph, shake the maraca."

Task Analysis:
1. Extend dominant arm downward toward handle of maraca (rattle), palm faced down.
2. Grasp handle of maraca with dominant hand using palmar grasp.
3. Bend elbow, raising maraca to chest level.
4. When beat is heard, flex wrist forward and downward away from body, shaking maraca downward to produce sound.
5. Immediately flex wrist inward and upward toward body, shaking maraca upward to produce sound, shaking maraca 1 time to beat.

6. Shake maraca second time to beat.
7. Shake maraca third time to beat.

Activity Guidelines/Special Adaptations:
1. If wrist is immobile, participant may shake the maraca (rattle) by waving entire arm at shoulder. Wrist straps can also be used to secure maraca to hand.
2. If participant has no use of upper limbs, he may place the maraca between teeth and shake head to shake maraca. Participant may also have maraca attached to a foot and he can move his foot to shake maraca to beat.
3. Maracas can be made using plastic containers filled with dried beans.
4. Initially the beat can be produced by the teacher clapping her hands together or, if there is one available, a metronome can be used. Eventually a record with an easily recognizable beat can be used.

Name of Activity: Play Tambourine

Instructional Objective: Given a tambourine, the participant will shake the tambourine 3 times, producing an audible sound, 80% of the time.
Materials: tambourine
Verbal Cue: "Ralph, shake the tambourine."

Task Analysis:
1. Grasp edge of tambourine with dominant hand using palmar grasp.
2. Raise tambourine to chest level by bending at elbow.
3. Raise nondominant hand, palm faced inward, to level parallel with tambourine by bending at elbow.
4. Position head of tambourine directly in front of and 4 inches away from palm of nondominant hand.
5. Strike head of tambourine against heel of nondominant hand by bending at elbow of dominant arm, shaking tambourine.
6. Shake tambourine second time.
7. Shake tambourine third time.

Activity Guidelines/Special Adaptations:
1. Participant can practice the movements necessary in this activity by using a frisbee or top of a cookie tin.
2. If participant has use of only one hand, the tambourine can be hit against the hip (this is often done by tampourine players, particularly when they are holding and singing into a microphone).
3. Harmonica playing if often recommended because it is a good exercise for the lungs. A device is available to hold the instrument in front of the player's mouth, leaving the hands free.

4. There is a deluxe rhythm band set available that includes tambourines, triangles, wrist bells, sand blocks, rhythm sticks, castanets, cymbals, and tom-tom and snare drums. There are enough pieces in the set to provide 15 to 25 people with instruments.

PET CARE

Name of Activity: Walk Dog on Leash

Instructional Objective; Given a dog, collar, and leash, the participant will put the leash and collar on the dog, and walk the dog 10 feet without letting go of the leash, 80% of the time.
Materials: dog, leash, collar
Verbal Cue: "Phyllis, put the leash on the dog and walk him/her."

Task Analysis:
1. Grasp ends of collar with both hands using pincer grasp.
2. Position collar directly above back of dog's neck.
3. Wrap collar around dog's neck by moving both hands downward toward each other.
4. Insert end of collar into one side of buckle.
5. Pull inserted collar end outward away from body by bending at elbow, until collar fits snugly around dog's neck.
6. Insert stem of buckle into hole in collar by extending thumb.
7. Insert end of collar into other side of buckle.
8. Grasp hook on end of leash with dominant hand using palmar grasp.
9. Open hook by sliding button backward with thumb.
10. Grasp ring on dog's collar with nondominant hand using pincer grasp.
11. Position open end of hook directly in front of edge of ring.
12. Slide open end of hook through edge of ring by moving hand sideways toward ring.
13. Release button on hook by extending fingers to close ring.
14. Release ring on collar by extending fingers.
15. Grasp looped end of leash with dominant hand using palmar grasp.
16. Allow leash to hang loosely by side while keeping a firm grasp on looped end of leash.
17. Walk 1 foot, allowing dog to stop when it desires.
18. Walk dog 2 feet.
19. Walk dog 4 feet.
20. Walk dog 6 feet.

21. Walk dog 8 feet.
22. Walk dog 10 feet.

Activity Guidelines/Special Adaptations:
1. Participants should practice this activity using a stuffed animal before attempting it on a real dog.
2. If manipulating the buckle on the collar is too difficult for participant, a collar can be made using Velcro strips or snaps to secure it around the dog's neck. Also, a chain collar that is simply looped over the dog's head may be easier to use.
3. A practice board with a hook and a buckle can be made for participants to practice this activity.
4. In order to make walking pleasurable for both the participant and the dog, the dog should have some basic leashtraining. This includes not straining or tugging at the leash (keeping pace with the person walking) and staying on one side of the person (so that the leash does not wrap around the legs).
5. Participant should accommodate dog's desire to stop along way.
6. Looped end of leash can be worn around wrist, bracelet-style, if participant has difficulty grasping.
7. Unusual pets, such as snakes, skunks, and raccoons, have a way of attracting other persons in the neighborhood. Pets are sometimes an excellent way of meeting and socializing with others.

Name of Activity: Feed Dog

Instructional Objective: Given a bag of dry dog food, a food scooper, and bowl, the participant will fill the bowl with dog food using the scoop, and feed the dog, 80% of the time.

Materials: dog, bag of dry dog food, food scoop, bowl
Verbal Cue: "Phyllis, feed the dog."

Task Analysis:
1. Grasp dog food scoop with dominant hand using palmar grasp.
2. Position scoop directly above opened bag of dog food.
3. Rotate wrist until open end of scoop is facing downward.
4. Lower scoop into bag by moving hand downward.
5. Push scoop into dog food by applying downward pressure onto scoop with hand, simultaneously rotating wrist until scoop is upright, filling scoop with dog food.
6. Raise scoop out of bag by moving hand upward.
7. Position scoop directly above center of dog food bowl.

8. Dump dog food into bowl by rotating wrist to invert scoop.
9. Continue scooping and dumping food into bowl until filled.
10. Release scoop onto table by lowering hand to table and extending fingers.
11. Grasp opposite sides of dog food bowl with both hands using palmar grasp.
12. Lower bowl to ground in front of dog by bending at knees.
13. Release bowl by extending fingers.

Activity Guidelines/Special Adaptations:
1. Initially the dog food bag can be opened before the activity begins. Eventually, the participant should be required to open and close the bag on her own.
2. A line can be painted on the inside of the bowl to indicate to participant when enough food is in the bowl. Also, individually wrapped portions of dog food are available that contain only the amount of dog food necessary for one meal.
3. Some dry dog foods require water to be added to them and this should be taken into consideration when choosing dog food. Also, while most dogs prefer canned food over dry, dry dog food is more economical and just as nutritious as canned.

Name of Activity: Use of Pooper-Scooper

Instructional Objective: Given a pooper-scooper and dog feces, the participant will use the pooper-scooper to pick up the feces, 80% of the time.
Materials: pooper-scooper, dog feces
Verbal Cue: "Phyllis, use the pooper-scooper."

Task Analysis:
1. Grasp handle of pooper-scooper with dominant hand using palmar grasp.
2. Extend dominant arm holding scooper downward to dog feces.
3. Position open end of scooper directly in front of dog feces.
4. Open scooper by depressing thumb on release switch.
5. Push scooper forward to contain dog feces in scooper pan.
6. Raise thumb from release switch to close scooper.
7. Lift scooper off ground by bending at elbow.
8. Walk to toilet.
9. Position pooper scooper directly above toilet bowl
10. Open scooper by depressing thumb on release switch.
11. Release feces into toilet by rotating wrist downward, dumping feces into toilet bowl.

Activity Guidelines/Special Adaptations:
1. Many pooper-scoopers have small shovel attachment for scooping dog excretion into scooper pan.
2. Participants can practice this activity using a dust pan or shovel. Pooper-scooper could be used with various objects to provide skill in function of scooper before attempting this activity.
3. The release button could be painted a bright color so that it is easily seen by participant.
4. The inclusion of this activity in teaching pet care is timely, considering the passage of laws in many cities that call for the levy of fines on those persons who do not clean up after their dogs.

PHOTOGRAPHY

Name of Activity: Use of Instamatic Camera

Instructional Objective: Given an Instamatic camera and a roll of film, the participant will insert the cartridge of film into the camera and take a photograph, 80% of the time.

Materials: instamatic camera, roll of film

Verbal Cue: "Leslie, take a picture of ___(name of person to be photographed)___."

Task Analysis:
1. Hold camera firmly in nondominant hand using palmar grasp (camera lens facing ground).
2. Place thumb of dominant hand on top of hinged back cover (note: location may differ on various cameras).
3. Depress latch to open hinged back cover by bending thumb downward.
4. Lower hinged back cover by rotating wrist away from camera.
5. Remove film cartridge from box and remove protective wrapping.
6. Hold cartridge in dominant hand using pincer grasp.
7. Position cartridge directly in front of and parallel with opened back of camera.
8. Insert cartridge into camera by pushing cartridge downward with fingertips.
9. Place fingers on outside of hinged back cover.
10. Press firmly against center of cover until it locks back into camera body.
11. Wind film advance to lock first exposure into place.
12. Look through camera.
13. Extend index finger of dominant hand.

14. Position index finger of dominant hand directly above shutter release button.
15. Bend index finger at second joint, applying downward pressure onto button until completely depressed.

Activity Guidelines/Special Adaptations:
1. A connecting wrist strap can be worn to eliminate the possibility of participant dropping the camera while loading the film into it.
2. The teacher can initially remove the film cartridge from its box and take off the protective wrapping before activity is implemented.
3. As a leadup activity, participant can practice placing different sized blocks into matching holes. This would be excellent practice for inserting film into a camera.
4. After first picture is taken, film advance must be wound to lock second exposure into place. When last picture has been shot, the film advance must be wound until it will not wind any more and black line appears in window.
5. Participant can initially practice using toilet paper roll or paper towel roll to look at an object. Ask participant to look at an object. Ask participant to look at several objects around the room and possibly name the objects as he sees them.
6. A Viewmaster could be used as a leadup activity to prepare participant to manipulate a real camera. The Viewmaster requires only that the participant look through the lens and point it toward a well lit area.
7. Larger handles could be attached to camera if participant has difficulty grasping.
8. When teaching the skill of turning head and hands toward specified objects, have participant make believe that the camera is glued to his face, resulting in simultaneous moving of head and camera.
9. Toy cameras that shoot water when the button is pressed can be reinforcing to participant and could be used as a leadup activity.
10. If there is more than one button on the camera, each button may be color-coded according to its function.
11. The button can be enlarged using adhesive tape to provide a better gripping surface. Textured adhesive tape will aid the participant in locating the button with his finger, rather than having to visually locate it.
12. Initially, this activity can be implemented using a camera without any film.
13. Participant should be taught to depress the button firmly yet gently, taking care to hold the camera steady.

14. The click of the shutter should serve as an indicator that button has been completely depressed.

Name of Activity: Make Photograph Album

Instructional Objective: Given a photograph album and 4 photographs, the participant will stick the photographs onto 1 page in the album, 80% of the time.

Materials: photograph album, 4 photographs

Verbal Cue: "Leslie, place the photographs in the album."

Task Analysis:
1. Take photographs with camera.
2. Bring finished cartridge to photo dealer or mail cartridge to developer.
3. Receive envelope containing developed photos.
4. Grasp cover of album with right hand using pincer grasp.
5. Open album to first page by moving cover to left side of body.
6. Grasp cellophane on top corner of first page with dominant hand using pincer grasp.
7. Peel cellophane backward off page by moving dominant hand downward toward bottom of album (sticky backing of page is now exposed).
8. Grasp first picture with dominant hand using pincer grasp.
9. Position picture directly above top left quarter of page.
10. Place picture onto page by lowering picture to page and extending fingers.
11. Place fingertips of dominant hand onto page.
12. Stick picture to page by applying downward pressure onto picture with fingertips.
13. Place remaining 3 pictures onto remaining quarters of first page.
14. Replace cellophane on pictures.

Activity Guidelines/Special Adaptations:
1. A larger than standard-sized photograph album can be used to increase the chance of success in placing the pictures on the page.
2. There are photograph albums available that do not have the sticky pages, but have sets of four tabs by which the four corners of the picture are held secure. Participants will find the album with the sticky pages easier to manipulate because it requires less manual dexterity.
3. Participants can use a photograph album to make several different kinds of collections (i.e., butterflies, leaves, baseball cards, etc.).

PLANT CARE

Name of Activity: Plant Seed

Instructional Objective: Given a flower pot, potting soil, spoon, and potting rocks, the participant will put the rocks and the potting soil in the pot, and plant the seed, 80% of the time.
Materials: flower pot, potting soil, potting rocks, spoon, newspaper, seed, pencil
Verbal Cue: "Elise, fill the flower pot with soil and plant a seed."

Task Analysis:
1. Kneel or sit opposite pot and soil.
2. Extend dominant hand downward to rocks, palm faced down.
3. Grasp handful of rocks with dominant hand using palmar grasp.
4. Position dominant hand holding rocks directly above pot.
5. Drop rocks into pot by extending fingers.
6. Continue filling pot with rocks until bottom is covered.
7. Grasp spoon with dominant hand using palmar grasp.
8. Position scoop end of spoon directly above open bag of potting soil.
9. Lower arm and spoon into soil by extending at elbow.
10. Raise arm up by bending at elbow, scooping soil with spoon.
11. Position spoon directly above pot.
12. Rotate wrist downward, emptying soil into pot.
13. Continue scooping and emptying soil into pot until it is filled to rim.
14. Extend dominant hand downward toward pencil, palm faced down.
15. Grasp pencil.
16. Position pencil directly above filled flower pot.
17. Lower pencil 3 inches into center of soil by extending at elbow.
18. Rotate pencil back and forth to form small hole in soil.
19. Raise pencil out of soil by bending at elbow.
20. Release pencil onto ground by extending fingers.
21. Extend dominant hand downward toward plant seed, palm faced down.
22. Grasp plant seed with dominant hand using pincer grasp.
23. Position seed directly above hole in soil.
24. Drop seed into hole by extending fingers.
25. Push top layer of soil into hole.
26. Pat top layer of soil down by applying gentle pressure onto soil with fingertips.

Activity Guidelines/Special Adaptations:
1. Since filling a pot with dirt can be somewhat messy, spreading layers of newspaper beneath the pot and soil will make cleanup easier.
2. Potting soil and pebbles are commercially available, but it is not

absolutely necessary to use them. Small rocks or pebbles can be gathered outside and soil from a garden can be used.
3. Tape or paint can be used on the inside of the pot to indicate rock level and soil level.
4. If participant has difficulty grasping a spoon, a larger spoon with the handle built up can be used, or a child's beach shovel would be handy. The participant can also use his or her hands to scoop the soil and fill the pot.
5. For participants having difficulty grasping seeds, place a single seed in small Dixie cup and have participant pour seed into flower pot.
6. Initially, seeds can be dumped onto aluminum tray, making it easier for participant to grasp a single seed.
7. Often, several seeds need to be planted in order to get one plant growing. Therefore, to increase chances for success, plant several seeds at one time.

Name of Activity: Water and Mist Plant

Instructional Objective: Given a water pitcher and a plant mister, the participant will water and mist a plant, 80% of the time.
Materials: water pitcher, plant mister, plant
Verbal Cue: "Elise, water and mist the plant."

Task Analysis:
1. Grasp handle of water pitcher with dominant hand using palmar grasp.
2. Raise spout of pitcher to level parallel with rim of pot by bending at elbow.
3. Rotate wrist counterclockwise, simultaneously moving spout toward center of pot, pouring $\frac{1}{2}$ inch of water onto top layer of soil (water will seep down to roots).
4. Grasp handle of plant mister with dominant hand using palmar grasp, placing thumb on trigger.
5. Apply downward pressure onto trigger with thumb, showering plant with spray of mist 1 time.
6. Continue misting plant until entire plant is misted.

Activity Guidelines/Special Adaptations:
1. A premeasured amount of water in a glass or cup can be used rather than a pitcher to eliminate the danger of overwatering. Continuous overwatering of a plant will rot the roots, so it is important to control not only the amount of water, but the frequency of watering.
2. Empty 409 or Windex bottles (that have been thoroughly cleaned) can be used instead of a commercial plant mister.

3. A plastic or styrofoam pitcher may be easier for some participants to grasp and lift.
4. It may be advisable to use plants requiring infrequent watering and misting to ensure success. A jade plant is an excellent choice, a wandering jew plant is attractive, yet requires minimal care. African violets are extremely sensitive.

SPECTATOR LEISURE/COMMUNITY EVENTS

Name of Activity: Go to Movie Theater

Instructional Objective: Given a neighborhood movie theater, the participant will attend the theater, 80% of the time.
Materials: movie theater, money for ticket
Verbal Cue: "Toby, let's go to the movies."

Task Analysis:
1. Purchase ticket.
2. Hand ticket to doorman.
3. Use vending machine or buy refreshment from vendor, if desired.
4. Locate seat.
5. Attend movie.
6. Leave movie theater.

Activity Guidelines/Special Adaptations:
1. This activity can be simulated in the classroom for practice. Many agencies and institutions provide movies for their residents; this would be an excellent opportunity to set up a simulated movie theater, complete with a ticket booth, doorman, refreshment stand, and seating arrangement. As participants become accustomed to the rituals involved in attending movies, these skills can be transferred to a real movie theater.
2. Persons in wheelchairs or on crutches should be encouraged to choose aisle seats near the rear of the theater.
3. Leaving a facility is just as important as entering; participants should be encouraged to wait courteously until there is an opening in the exiting stream of people.

Name of Activity: Attend Social Dance

Instructional Objective: Given a social dance event, the participant will attend the dance, 80% of the time.
Materials: dance hall, social dance event.
Verbal Cue: "Toby, let's go to the dance."

Task Analysis:
1. Enter dance facility.
2. Purchase ticket or pay for admission if necessary.
3. Choose a dance partner.
4. Walk up to prospective dance partner.
5. Request a dance by asking, "Would you like to dance?" or manually by pointing at dance partner and self, then to dance floor.
   a) If answer is yes, escort partner to dance floor.
   b) If answer is no, say "Thank you" and walk away.
6. Say "Thank you" to partner after every dance.
7. Continue requesting dances and dancing with desired partner(s) until music stops and dance event is over.
8. Leave dance hall.

Activity Guidelines/Special Adaptations:
1. This activity can be simulated in the classroom for practice. A record player can be used to provide music and participants can practice requesting a dance and thanking the partner when the dance is over.
2. In this age of liberation, female participants should be encouraged to request dances with males. Particularly shy males will not only feel flattered, but may eventually integrate and use the correct procedure when requesting a dance with future partners.
3. Refreshments are usually available for thirsty dancers; offering to get a refreshment for a dance partner is an important social aspect of attending dances and should be encouraged.
4. Instruction incorporating the art of social chit-chat can be included in conjunction with this activity. Exchanging names and places of residence, hobbies, etc. can be encouraged.
5. Many communities periodically hold dances for handicapped individuals. These are often joyous social events for handicapped persons, even if only as spectators. Dances are not only socially reinforcing, but socially enriching, and should be part of every person's life, handicapped and nonhandicapped alike.

SPECTATOR LEISURE/HOME

Name of Activity: Use of Record Player

Instructional Objective: Given a record player and an LP record, the participant will listen to the record, 80% of the time.
Materials: record player, LP record
Verbal Cue: "Wayne, play a record."

Task Analysis:
1. Extend dominant hand downward to desired record album.
2. Grasp record with dominant hand using palmar grasp.
3. Pull record out of case by bending at elbow.
4. Position nondominant hand directly below open side of record album, palm faced up.
5. Rotate both wrists so that record slides out of album cover onto open palm of nondominant hand.
6. Grasp record album with nondominant hand using palmar grasp.
7. Grasp record on opposite edges of record with both hands using pincer grasp.
8. Position hole of record directly above spindle in center of turntable.
9. Lower record onto turntable by extending at elbows, sliding spindle through hole in record.
10. Release record by extending fingers.
11. Position dominant index finger directly above automatic button (that automatically moves arm over to record and lowers needle onto record).
12. Push button to activate record player.

Activity Guidelines/Special Adaptations:
1. Initially, records can be stored without the album covers, eliminating the need for participant to remove record from jacket.
2. Records should be stored vertically to allow easy grasping by participant (it is also better for records to be stored this way). A storage container can be constructed out of wood or cardboard. Wooden crates can be obtained from grocery stores and are excellent for storing records.
3. Initially, place a favorite record of the participant in the storage case. Perhaps it could be marked with a brightly colored piece of paper.
4. A listening center in the classroom can be arranged and a specific time for music listening set aside each day.
5. Most turntables have automatic buttons that are pressed or manipulated in order to automatically place needle arm on the record.
6. An extended level could be attached to the arm or to the automatic button of the record player for participants who have difficulty grasping.
7. Some turntables have a cueing device if there is no automatic button. The arm is positioned over the record and the needle gently lowered onto the record by use of the cue. This would eliminate scratching the records by participants who have poor muscle control.

Name of Activity: Use of Television

Instructional Objective: Given a television set, the participant will turn on the television and select a desired program, 80% of the time.
Materials: television set
Verbal Cue: "Wayne, turn on the TV."

Task Analysis:
1. Extend dominant hand to on/off knob.
2. Grasp knob with dominant hand using pincer grasp.
3. Turn TV on by rotating wrist clockwise to turn knob or by bending elbow to pull knob outward toward body.
4. Rotate wrist clockwise or counterclockwise to adjust volume to comfortable level.
5. Grasp channel selector with dominant hand using palmar grasp.
6. Rotate wrist clockwise until desired channel and/or picture appears.

Activity Guidelines/Special Adaptations:
1. The channel numbers received in a particular locale can be marked with a bright color on the channel selector to aid participant in knowing which channels (numbers) can be received on the television set.
2. Arrows can be used on the on/off knob to indicate the direction in which to turn or pull the knob for power and volume.
3. Some participants may be unable to grasp the small on/off knob or the channel selector; a remote control device is available that requires the participant to push buttons rather than grasp and turn knobs.
4. Although television viewing can be considered somewhat of a national pastime, this activity should not be encouraged as the sole leisure time activity.

SUNBATHING

Name of Activity: Putting on Bathing Suit

Instructional Objective: Given a bathing suit, the participant will put it on, 80% of the time.
Materials: bathing suit
Verbal Cue: "Becky, put on the bathing suit."

Task Analysis:
1. Grasp sides of bathing suit with both hands using palmar grasp.
2. Bend at knees, lowering body into chair, assuming sitting position.
3. Lower bottom of bathing suit to floor by bending forward at waist.
4. Position right foot directly above right leg hole of suit.

5. Lower foot through hole to floor by extending leg at knee.
6. Place left leg through left leg hole.
7. Raise suit upward on legs by raising body upright at waist.
8. Fully extend legs at knees and assume standing position.
9. Pull suit upward to waist by bending arms at elbows (*males* putting on bathing suit).
10. Position right hand directly above right arm hole of suit.
11. Place arm through hole by extending arm at elbow.
12. Grasp right side of suit with left hand using palmar grasp.
13. Pull right side of suit up onto right shoulder by bending left arm at elbow.
14. Place left arm through left arm hole of suit.
15. Pull left side of suit up onto left shoulder with right hand, (females putting on bathing suit).

Activity Guidelines/Special Adaptations:
1. Participant should be taught to look for tag on inside of bathing suit that will indicate the back of the suit.
2. For male participants, a bathing suit with an elasticized waist band, or a velcro waist band, will be the least difficult to put on. For female participants, a one-piece bathing suit will be the easiest to put on.
3. Have participant lie on floor if muscular coordination limits self-standing or sitting. Participant can also lean against a wall for balance if needed.
4. Participant can be encouraged to wear bathing suit to beach or swimming pool, instead of dressing at facility's bath house. Familiar surroundings and comfort of home will simplify process.

Name of Activity: Put on Suntan Lotion

Instructional Objective: Given a bottle of suntan lotion, the participant will rub the suntan lotion on her body, covering at least arms and legs, 80% of the time.

Materials: suntan lotion

Verbal Cue: "Becky, put on suntan lotion."

Task Analysis:
1. Extend dominant arm downward to bottle of suntan lotion.
2. Grasp suntan lotion bottle with dominant hand using palmar grasp.
3. Grasp cap of bottle with nondominant hand using pincer grasp.
4. Unscrew bottle cap by rotating wrist counterclockwise.
5. Release bottle cap by extending fingers.
6. Position nondominant hand at chest level, palm faced up, fingers extended.

Hobbies 123

7. Position bottle directly above nondominant palm.
8. Rotate dominant wrist until spout of bottle is directly above nondominant palm.
9. Apply inward pressure between fingers of dominant hand to squeeze small amount (size of a quarter) of lotion onto palm.
10. Move nondominant hand with lotion to dominant arm by bending at elbow until palm makes contact with arm.
11. Move hand against arm in a circular motion, rubbing lotion into skin.
12. When lotion in palm has been rubbed into skin, squeeze more lotion onto palm.
13. Continue rubbing lotion into all exposed areas of skin.

Activity Guidelines/Special Adaptations:
1. A circle the size of a quarter can be painted on the participant's palms with washable ink to indicate an adequate amount of lotion to be squeezed into palm each time.
2. The teacher may initially loosen the cap on the bottle, making it easier to remove. A jar or tube of suntan lotion, having a larger cap, may be easier for some participants to manipulate. There are also aerosol containers available that dispense a fine spray of suntan lotion by pushing a trigger. These should be used with caution, however.
3. If participant has use of only one hand, she could hold the bottle between her knees to unscrew the cap. Lotion could be applied directly to the body from the bottle and rubbed in with the functional hand.

TABLE GAME HOBBIES

Name of Activity: Play Foosball

Instructional Objective: Given a Foosball table and another player, the participant will manipulate his two rows of playing men to hit the ball into his opponent's goal to score a point (first to score 7 points wins game), 80% of the time.
Materials: Foosball table, money
Verbal Cue: "Tom, play Foosball."

Task Analysis:
1. Stand directly in front of coin slot of machine.
2. Grasp coin with dominant hand using pincer grasp.
3. Raise coin to level parallel with coin slot by bending elbow of dominant arm.
4. Position edge of coin directly in front of coin slot.
5. Push coin into slot by extending at elbow.

6. Release coin by extending fingers.
7. Stand facing levers on side of Foosball table.
8. Grasp levers with both hands using palmar grasp.
9. Follow path of ball across table.
10. Position one row of playing men directly in path of ball by either extending or bending at either elbow, pushing or pulling appropriate lever to move row of men laterally across table.
11. When ball makes contact with playing man and has been stopped, quickly rotate either wrist counterclockwise to turn appropriate lever, causing playing man to make contact with ball, hitting ball forward toward opponent's goal.
12. Opponent attempts to block ball.
13. Hit ball into goal, scoring one point.
14. Continue playing until one player scores 7 points to win the game.

Activity Guidelines/Special Adaptations:
1. Initially, give the participant the proper amount of change needed to operate the machine. Many machines use only quarters to operate and will not take combinations of coins.
2. Instruction in recognition of coin denominations can be incorporated into this activity.
3. Simulate coin insertion of various machines by constructing cardboard coins for instructional purposes. Some machines have coin slots, others have levers that slide coin into machine.
4. Levers can be built up using adhesive tape or sponge to provide a better gripping surface for participant.
5. For participants in wheelchairs, the table can be lowered to a comfortable level and the levers can be elongated by attaching wooden dowels to them.
6. A participant having use of only one hand can still play Foosball by using one hand to alternately manipulate the two rows of playing men.
7. Initially, a heavier ball of the same size as the Foosball can be used to slow the pace of the game, making it easier for participants to move the ball around the table.
8. Since all 4 levers extend outward on both sides of the table, with proficiency, 4 players can play; 2 players manipulating 2 levers on each side of the table.

Name of Activity: Play Pinball

Instructional Objective: Given a pinball machine, the participant will release 3 balls, one at a time, and manipulate the flippers to score points before the ball goes out of play, 80% of the time.

Materials: pinball machine
Verbal Cue: "Tom, play pinball."

Task Analysis:
1. Stand directly in front of and facing pinball machine.
2. Place left hand on flipper button on left side of machine by extending arm outward.
3. Position first and second fingers of left hand on button.
4. Grasp ball release lever with right hand using palmar grasp.
5. Pull lever completely out by bending right arm at elbow.
6. Extend fingers, releasing lever, causing ball to be released into scoring area.
7. Position right hand on right flipper button.
8. Follow path of ball across scoring area.
9. When ball approaches flippers, push buttons by bending fingers inward toward machine, causing flippers to hit the ball upward into scoring area.
10. Continue manipulating flippers to keep ball in scoring area until ball rolls past flippers and is out of play.
11. Release second ball.
12. Manipulate flippers to keep second ball in scoring area until ball rolls past flippers and is out of play.
13. Release third ball.

Activity Guidelines/Special Adaptations:
1. Pinball is reinforcing for all players because points are automatically scored as ball travels across scoring area. Even a player who is initially unable to operate flippers adequately can still enjoy releasing ball and watching it ricochet across table with resulting flashing lights and bells.
2. There are small, portable pinball machines for use at home or school that do not require money to operate. Participants can practice on these machines before attempting to operate commercial pinball machine. Also, portable pinball machines can be positioned at level accessible to participant in wheelchair.
3. Flipper buttons can be painted bright colors or covered with adhesive tape.

Name of Activity: Play Electric Bowling

Instructional Objective: Given an electric bowling game, the participant will shoot his bowling disc toward the target, attempting to knock down as many pins as possible, 80% of the time.
Materials: electric bowling game
Verbal Cue: "Tom, play the bowling game."

Task Analysis:
1. Stand facing bowling machine.
2. Grasp bowling disc in dominant hand using palmar grasp.
3. Position disc at starting line on table, directly in line with center pin.
4. Quickly push disc forward along table toward pins by extending at elbow.
5. When elbow is fully extended, release disc by extending fingers, causing disc to move toward pins.
6. Continue shooting disc toward pins until game is over.

Activity Guidelines/Special Adaptations:
1. When disc is thrown toward target, it is automatically rebounded back along table to starting line where participant retrieves it and shoots again. Game is over when pins can no longer be knocked down and score no longer registers when disc is thrown.
2. This game can be played alone or with opponent, each player taking alternate shots with disc.
3. There are variations on most electric bowling games ranging from simple (merely aiming the disc at pins and shooting) to complex (participant must time shot to coincide with flashing light to score).
4. Electric bowling can be played even by participants lacking good motor coordination since sides of table make it almost impossible for disc to leave playing area.

Name of Activity: Play Pool

Instructional Objective: Given a pool table, cue stick, rack of balls, and another player, the participant will hit one group of designated balls (i.e., striped or solid) into table pockets by hitting cue ball (white) first each time, 50% of the time.

Materials: regulation pool table, balls, cue stick

Verbal Cue: "Tom, play pool."

Task Analysis:
1. Stand facing pool table opposite ball formation (cue ball placed near participant opposite center ball of formation).
2. Grasp larger end of cue stick with dominant hand using palmar grasp.
3. Bend fingers of nondominant hand to make fist.
4. Extend thumb of nondominant hand horizontally.
5. Place fist on table opposite ball formation by lowering hand to table.
6. Place tip of cue stick between thumb and fist of nondominant hand.
7. Align tip of cue stick with cue ball and racked balls.
8. Quickly extend dominant arm at elbow to strike cue ball with tip of cue stick, breaking up ball formation with impact of cue ball.

9. Locate one of participant's designated balls that is situated between cue ball and pocket.
10. Position body directly behind cue ball and opposite pocket.
11. Strike cue ball with tip of cue stick, driving cue ball into middle ball, causing middle ball to hit into pocket with impact of cue ball.
12. Continue shooting designated balls into pockets with cue ball until all designated balls have been hit into pockets.

Activity Guidelines/Special Adaptations:
1. Bumper pool is a good leadup activity to playing regulation pool. The table is smaller and the balls are hit directly into the holes, rather than using the cue ball to sink another ball.
2. Cue sticks come in various sizes and should be chosen for comfort. Generally, smaller persons use a smaller, lighter cue stick that is easier to manipulate.
3. If participant has difficulty holding a cue stick, the end of the stick that is held (the thicker end) can be built up using foam rubber or textured adhesive tape. The lower part of the stick (the thinner end) must be smooth so that it can slide easily over the fingers.
4. All community pool centers have a wooden adapted device, a bridge. This is used by even the best players to make difficult shots, when ball cannot be reached with cue stick alone. It is, in reality, an extension of player's arm—cue stick rests on bridge just as it normally rests on player's nondominant hand. A bridge is an excellent adaptation for those participants lacking adequate eye-hand coordination or fine motor control, since it steadies cue stick and lines up stick accurately with ball.
5. Initially, teacher can stand directly behind participant and hold cue stick along with participant, physically guiding participant through motion of aiming and shooting.
6. Whether player shoots striped or solid balls depends upon person who breaks ball formation with cue ball; if ball is hit into pocket on break, that ball (either striped or solid) represents balls that will be shot by player for remainder of game. If no ball is hit into pocket on break, other player then has choice of hitting either striped or solid balls.
7. Rather than designating certain balls to certain players, a game can consist of two players taking turns shooting at any ball. The number of balls shot in pockets by each player can be scored.
8. Cue sticks with wrist straps can be provided to aid with grip control.
9. Regular wooden pool bridge can be used by participant confined to wheelchair.
10. A spring loaded billiard cue is available (it was designed by a high

level quadriplegic). Made of lightweight aluminum, it requires pushing a button to release spring loaded shaft; button can be triggered by thumb, hand, arm, chin, etc.
11. An adjustable pool table, available from the J. L. Hammett Co., is excellent for those participants in wheelchairs.
12. A small pool table with automatic ball return, 2-player scorer, and spring-action cue sticks would be good leadup activity. It is small enough to be placed on table top and can be used to teach participants rules and strategies for pool.

Chapter 7
SPORTS

While accepting the idea that sports, especially vigorous, high energy activities are for everyone, in the past it was typically recognized as a recreational pursuit in which only males excelled. Today however, females, young and old, disabled, and nondisabled are active participants in sports. Sports activity can provide constructive and rewarding experiences for athletes and spectators. There are team sports (e.g., softball, volleyball), and dual sports (e.g., bowling, shuffleboard), as well as individual ones (e.g., fishing, jogging). The sports activity area, sometimes referred to as physical recreation, includes leisure activities of a gross motor nature and usually requires a relatively large amount of energy exertion. Participation in sports events provides opportunities to develop specific motor skills that are necessary for a healthy life. Not only can the participant practice competition, and learn to play within the rules and structure of the activity, but he or she can also learn about social interaction, concentration, and setting goals for self-improvement. Individuals should be given the opportunity to participate in a variety of sports and perform with greater skill and technique as they mature. With increasing participation in active and spectator sports by all segments of the population, sports have become an integral part of our culture.

The sports skills in this chapter include:

Age Level*	Sports Skills	Page
	BADMINTON	
C/A	Underhand Shot	130
C/A	Overhand Shot	131
C/A	Serve	132
	BASKETBALL	
C/A	Shoot Basketball	133
C/A	Dribble Basketball	134
	BOWLING	
C/A	Select Bowling Ball	135
C/A	Roll Ball Down Alley	136
C	Reposition Pins (Toy Set)	137
	FISHING	
C/A	Bait Hook	138
C/A	Cast Baited Fishing Line	139
C/A	Catch A Fish	140
	HANDBALL	
C/A	Put On Glove	141
C/A	Serve Handball	142
C/A	Hit Ball Against Wall	143

* C, Indicates chronologically age-appropriate for child; A, Indicates chronologically age-appropriate for adolescent and adult; C/A, Indicates chronologically age-appropriate for child, adolescent, and adult.

	JOGGING	
C/A	Arm-Leg Rotation	143
	PLAYGROUND EQUIPMENT	
C	See-Saw Play	144
C	Sliding Board Play	145
C	Swing Play	147
	SHUFFLEBOARD	
C/A	Line Up Discs	148
C/A	Shoot Disc	149
	SOFTBALL	
C/A	Underhand Throw	149
C/A	Catch Ball	150
C/A	Hit Ball	151
	SWIMMING	
C/A	Enter Swimming Pool	152
C/A	Walk Through Water	153
C/A	Breath Control	154
	VOLLEYBALL	
C/A	Underhand Serve	155
C/A	Return Ball Over Net	156
	WEIGHTLIFTING	
C/A	Curl	157
C/A	Lift Weight Over Head . . .	158
	WINTER SPORTS	
C/A	Make Snowball	158
C/A	Sledding	159

BADMINTON

Name of Activity: Underhand Shot

Instructional Objective: Given a badminton racket, a birdie, and a net 5 feet away, the participant will hit the birdie over the net, 80% of the time.

Materials: badminton racket, birdie, net

Verbal Cue: "Margie, hit the birdie over the net"

Task Analysis:
1. Extend dominant arm downward toward handle of racket, palm faced down (handle of racket facing dominant side of body).
2. Lower dominant arm until palm makes contact with handle of racket 3 inches from bottom.
3. Curl fingers around outer edge of handle.
4. Wrap thumb around opposite side of handle.
5. Apply inward pressure between thumb and fingers to grasp handle firmly.
6. Bend elbow, lifting racket to waist level.
7. Rotate wrist clockwise so that face of racket is perpendicular to ground.

8. Follow flight of birdie through air.
9. Position face of racket directly below approaching birdie.
10. At point of contact with birdie, quickly extend elbow, raising racket upward and outward toward net, hitting birdie 1 foot.
11. Hit birdie 2 feet.
12. Hit birdie 3 feet.
13. Hit birdie 4 feet.
14. Hit birdie 5 feet over net.

Activity Guidelines/Special Adaptations:
1. Any racket may be used; a racket with a short handle will be easier for beginning players to hold and swing.
2. The handle of the racket may be made larger for easier grasping by wrapping it with sponge and tape or with foam rubber.
3. The participant may stand 3 feet away from the net to ensure a more proficient shot. As the participant becomes more accurate, the distance from the net may be increased.

Name of Activity: Overhand shot

Instructional Objective: Given a badminton racket, a birdie, and a net 5 feet away, the participant will hit the birdie over the net, 80% of the time.
Materials: badminton racket, birdie, net
Verbal Cue: "Margie, hit the birdie over the net."

Task Analysis:
1. Hold racket.
2. Follow flight of birdie through air.
3. Bend elbow, raising racket to head level, face of racket parallel to net.
4. Extend elbow, raising racket upward 6 inches.
5. Bend wrist backward 45°, tilting racket backward.
6. At point of contact with birdie, quickly extend elbow, moving racket upward and outward, hitting birdie 1 foot.
7. Hit birdie 2 feet.
8. Hit birdie 3 feet.
9. Hit birdie 4 feet.
10. Hit birdie 5 feet over net.

Activity Guidelines/Special Adaptations:
1. Game should be taught indoors since the birdie's light weight can make its path subject to slight breezes therefore more difficult to follow. Heavier birdies can also be used to stabilize the movement.
2. A large yarn ball can be substituted for the birdie. The yarn ball is easier to locate when hit in the air and is easier to hit with the racket.

3. Larger badminton rackets are made with face diameters almost 1½ times as large as a standard racket. These rackets can initially be used with participants until they become more proficient and can handle a regulation racket.

Name of Activity: Serve

Instructional Objective: Given a badminton racket, a birdie, and a net 5 feet away, the participant will serve the birdie over the net, 80% of the time.
Materials: badminton racket, net, birdie
Verbal Cue: "Margie, serve the birdie over the net."

Task Analysis:
1. Hold racket.
2. Extend nondominant arm upward toward birdie lying on face of racket, palm faced down, thumb and index finger extended.
3. Lower nondominant arm until thumb and index finger make contact with opposite sides of open end of birdie.
4. Apply inward pressure between thumb and index finger to grasp birdie firmly.
5. Bend elbow of nondominant arm, raising birdie to shoulder level.
6. Bend elbow of dominant arm, raising racket parallel to net.
7. Extend elbow of dominant arm, raising racket upward 6 inches.
8. Bend wrist backward 45°, tilting racket backward.
9. Extend nondominant elbow, positioning birdie 6 inches away from body at eye level.
10. Quickly raise nondominant arm upward at shoulder, simultaneously extending thumb and index finger, releasing birdie into air above head.
11. Follow flight of birdie in air.
12. As birdie descends, extend dominant elbow, moving racket upward and outward toward birdie, making contact with birdie and hitting it forward 1 foot.
13. Hit birdie 2 feet.
14. Hit birdie 3 feet.
15. Hit birdie 4 feet.
16. Hit birdie 5 feet over net, serving birdie.

Activity Guidelines/Special Adaptations:
1. After the participants have mastered the component skills or during the time they are learning the skills, a team game may be introduced. Team games, in addition to teaching the component skills required to play the game, can teach spatial awareness through position play.

Playing a particular position on the court and rotating from position to position reinforces the concepts of right, left, center, front, and back. Starting with a small number of persons on a team and gradually increasing the number of team members is educationally sound, whereas assigning 8 to 10 persons to a team is not. Socially, children must learn to relate to and work with 1 or 2 friends before participating in larger impersonal games.
2. Participant may serve standing 1 foot from net instead of from the regulation serving position. Gradually increase distance from the net until participant reaches criterion.

BASKETBALL

Name of Activity: Shoot Basketball

Instructional Objective: Given a basketball and a basketball hoop 3 feet away, the participant will shoot the ball into the basket, 25% of the time.
Materials: basketball, basketball hoop
Verbal Cue: "Mark, shoot the ball into the basket."

Task Analysis:
1. Stand directly behind basketball, 3 feet away from and facing basketball hoop, feet parallel and 6 inches apart.
2. Bend knees, lowering body toward ground.
3. Bend forward at waist 45°.
4. Extend arms outward toward opposite sides of ball, palms faced inward.
5. Move arms inward at shoulders until palms make contact with sides of ball.

Activity Guidelines/Special Adaptations:
1. Height and diameter of basketball hoop may be adjusted to suit ability level of participants (e.g., basket may be lowered to shoulder height or lower; Hula Hoop or large trashcan may be used for a wider basket.)
2. Initially, participant can stand fairly close to basket (3 feet); with proficiency, he should move further away from the basket until he is shooting from the foul line. Shooting from the foul line should be encouraged (if participant has the ability), as this is an important part of the game.

Name of Activity: Dribble Basketball

Instructional Objective: Given a basketball, the participant will dribble the ball 3 consecutive times, 80% of the time.

Materials: basketball

Verbal Cue: "Mark, dribble the ball."

Task Analysis:
1. Stand directly behind basketball, feet parallel and 6 inches apart.
2. Bend knees, lowering body toward ground.
3. Bend forward at waist 45°.
4. Extend arms outward toward opposite sides of ball, palms faced inward.
5. Move arms inward at shoulders until palms make contact with sides of ball.
6. Apply inward pressure between hands to grasp ball firmly.
7. Bend elbows, bringing ball to waist.
8. Extend knees, raising body to upright position.
9. Quickly extend elbows downward, simultaneously extending fingers, applying downward pressure onto ball with hands, releasing ball to ground, causing it to bounce 1 time.
10. As ball ascends to waist level, position dominant hand directly above top of ball, palm faced down, fingers extended.
11. At point of contact with ball, quickly extend elbow downward, applying downward pressure onto ball with hand causing ball to bounce second time, dribbling basketball 1 time.
12. Dribble basketball second time.
13. Dribble basketball third time.

Activity Guidelines/Special Adaptations:
1. Depending on the conditions and degree of eye-hand coordination, the basketball can be made livelier by adding more air to it, or it may be slightly deflated to slow the ball down, making dribbling easier.
2. A larger ball (e.g., beach ball) may be used for participants having problems controlling the ball.
3. A player may be allowed to take as many steps as he needs without dribbling in a game situation.
4. A player may be allowed to dribble with both hands even though the rule states the one-handed dribble.
5. If participant is unable to strike the ball with his palm, he can use a paddle attached to his dominant hand to dribble the ball.
6. Although dribbling the ball is an important skill to acquire when learning to play basketball, the participant should initially be encouraged to practice bouncing and catching the basketball. Passing

the ball to another player in this manner (bouncing) is a maneuver often used in basketball games.
7. As participant becomes more proficient in bouncing and catching the basketball, games can be played in which the participants pass the ball to each other by bouncing it rather than throwing it.
8. Have participants stand in a circle and bounce the ball to a player in the circle after calling aloud the name of the player to whom the ball is bounced. Standing in a circle will also confine the ball in a small area, eliminating the need to chase a missed ball. This type of game is also excellent for improving eye-hand coordination as well as exercising auditory attendance.
9. Encourage participants to catch the ball no higher than chest level, where they can have maximum control of the ball.

BOWLING

Name of Activity: Select Bowling Ball

Instructional Objective: Given 2 bowling balls of different weights, the participant will choose a ball that she can place her fingers into and lift easily, 80% of the time.
Materials: 2 bowling balls of different weights
Verbal Cue: "Cindy, pick a bowling ball."

Task Analysis:
1. Extend dominant arm downward toward holes in bowling ball, palm faced down, fingers extended.
2. Rotate wrist forward 90° so that fingers are pointing downward toward ground.
3. Lower dominant arm until fingers are positioned directly above holes in ball.
4. Position thumb directly above largest hole in ball.
5. Position middle finger directly above hole to left of thumb.
6. Position ring finger directly above hole to right of thumb.
7. Extend elbow downward, lowering fingers into holes, index finger and pinky finger extended and resting on top of ball. (If fingers do not easily fit into holes, repeat steps 1–7 with second ball.)
8. Extend nondominant arm outward toward bottom of ball, palm faced up, fingers extended.
9. Raise nondominant arm upward at shoulder until palm makes contact with ball.
10. Bend elbow of dominant arm, raising ball off rack, simultaneously

moving nondominant arm inward at shoulder, sliding nondominant hand under ball to support ball as it is lifted.

Activity Guidelines/Special Adaptations:
1. Small children and those lacking sufficient arm strength should use lighter balls. Balls are available in 10–16 pound weights that have a handle grip that will automatically return flush to the ball when released. The handle will never catch fingers. This may be used for participants having difficulty lifting a conventional ball with holes.
2. For participants having extreme difficulty lifting, a Nerf bowling ball or a lightweight plastic bowling ball may be used with a toy set (obviously, it could not be used in a community bowling alley).
3. In a community bowling alley, the solid black balls are usually the heavier ones and the multicolored or starred balls are the 8–10 pound ones.
4. Choice of balls should initially be minimal; add more balls gradually to the selection.

Name of Activity: Roll Ball Down Alley

Instructional Objective: Given a bowling ball and a set of 10 bowling pins, the participant will roll the ball down the alley toward the pins, knocking down at least 1 pin, 80% of the time.
Materials: bowling ball, set of 10 bowling pins
Verbal Cue: "Cindy, roll the ball."

Task Analysis:
1. Pick up ball from ball return.
2. Stand facing pins, feet parallel and 6 inches apart.
3. Approach foul line.
4. Pivot dominant arm holding ball forward at shoulder, swinging ball forward toward pins in a pendulum motion.
5. When elbow is fully extended, extend fingers of dominant hand, releasing ball, causing ball to roll down alley, knocking down at least 1 pin.

Activity Guidelines/Special Adaptations:
1. Participants without use of arms can use feet to roll or push the ball down the alley.
2. Nonambulatory persons in wheelchairs should face the pins squarely and take two or more preliminary swings before releasing the ball.
3. Physically handicapped participants can use a tubular steel bowling ball ramp to guide ball down alley. Some persons can remove the ball from the ball return and place it on the ramp unassisted. Then the ramp can be positioned to aim for different pins.

4. The participants can practice rolling a ball to each other on a carpeted floor as a leadup skill to rolling a bowling ball down an alley. Initially, the distance between the participants should be short and increased with proficiency on part of participants.
5. With all these adapted devices available, even the most severely handicapped individual can learn to enjoy bowling.

Name of Activity: Reposition Pins (If Toy Set is Used)

Instructional Objective: Given 10 numbered, plastic bowling pins and a numbered floor diagram of proper pin placement, the participant will set up the pins for bowling, 80% of the time.
Materials: 10 plastic, numbered bowling pins, numbered floor diagram
Verbal Cue: "Cindy, set up the bowling pins."

Task Analysis:
1. Extend dominant arm downward toward #1 pin, palm faced inward.
2. Move dominant arm inward at shoulder until palm makes contact with neck of pin.
3. Curl fingers around neck of pin.
4. Wrap thumb around opposite side of neck of pin.
5. Apply inward pressure between thumb and fingers to grasp pin firmly.
6. Position #1 pin directly above the number 1 painted on the bottom point of the triangular floor marking.
7. Lower arm until bottom of pin makes contact with floor.
8. Extend fingers, releasing pin onto ground in upright position.
9. Pick up #2 pin.
10. Position #2 pin directly above the number 2 painted on floor marking.
11. Lower arm until bottom of pin makes contact with floor.
12. Extend fingers, releasing pin onto ground in upright position.
13. Place #3 pin on number 3 on floor.
14. Place #4 pin on floor.
15. Place #5 pin on floor.
16. Place #6 pin on floor.
17. Place #7 pin on floor.
18. Place #8 pin on floor.
19. Place #9 pin on floor.
20. Place #10 pin on floor, completing the repositioning of pins.

Activity Guidelines/Special Adaptations:
1. A handle may be placed on top of pins to make grasping easier.
2. Initially, it would be helpful to paint or tape numbers on the pins

corresponding to numbers printed on a floor diagram showing the proper placement of pins. The numbers can gradually be phased out as the participant learns the positioning of the pins, and eventually the floor marker can be eliminated.
3. "Five Pins" is a commercial game available in which pins do not need to be picked up after each shot. This game may be used if participant is not able to grasp and pick up pins after knocking them down.
4. Foam bowling pins are available for use with a playground ball. Their large width and light weight makes them desirable for use with persons having difficulty grasping and/or who have limited arm strength.

FISHING

Name of Activity: Bait Hook

Instructional Objective: Given an earthworm (bait) and a fishhook, the participant will bait the hook, 80% of the time.
Materials: fishhook, earthworm (bait)
Verbal Cue: "Kathy, put the worm on the hook."

Task Analysis:
1. Extend nondominant arm downward toward bait bucket, palm faced down, thumb and index finger extended.
2. Lower nondominant arm until thumb and index finger make contact with opposite sides of earthworm.
3. Apply inward pressure between thumb and index finger to grasp earthworm firmly.
4. Bend elbow, raising worm to chest level.
5. Extend dominant arm downward toward fishhook, palm faced down, thumb and index finger extended.
6. Lower dominant arm until thumb and index finger make contact with opposite sides of curved end of hook.
7. Apply inward pressure between thumb and index finger to grasp hook firmly.
8. Bend elbow, raising hook to chest level.
9. Position point of hook directly below body of worm.
10. Keeping worm stationary, raise dominant arm upward at shoulder, pushing point of hook through worm.
11. Extend fingers of nondominant hand, releasing worm onto hook.

Activity Guidelines/Special Adaptations:
1. Initially, a wire pipe cleaner can be bent into the shape of a fishing hook and elbow macaroni can be used to replace the bait (earthworm).

Have participants practice sliding the macaroni onto the pipe cleaner until they are skilled in manipulating the hook. After a substantial period of practice with the substitutes, genuine fishhooks and worms may be utilized.
2. Larger hooks can initially be used, making it easier for participant to manipulate the hook. Obviously, larger hooks have sharper and larger points. A wire clipper can be used to clip the end of the hook, thereby reducing the danger of getting stuck with the point. Even with the point cut off, a worm can still be pushed onto the hook.
3. Back part of fishhook can be built up by twisting a pipe cleaner around it.
4. Rubber worms and rubber flies, instead of real worms, can be used to bait the hook.

Name of Activity: Cast Baited Fishing Line

Instructional Objective: Given a pole with a line and a baited hook, the participant will cast the line 5 feet into the water, 80% of the time.

Materials: fishing rod, fishing line, fishhook baited with worm, fishing area

Verbal Cue: "Kathy, throw your line into the water."

Task Analysis:
1. Stand 2 feet away from and facing water, feet parallel and 6 inches apart.
2. Bend knees, lowering body toward ground.
3. Extend dominant arm outward toward pole, palm faced down, fingers extended.
4. Lower dominant arm until palm makes contact with pole 1 foot from bottom end.
5. Curl fingers around pole.
6. Wrap thumb around opposite side of pole.
7. Apply inward pressure between thumb and fingers to grasp pole firmly.
8. Bend elbow, bringing pole to waist level.
9. Extend knees, raising body to upright position.
10. Rotate wrist 90° clockwise so that pole is perpendicular to front of body, parallel to ground.
11. Extend elbow fully to dominant side of body, bringing pole to side.
12. Rotate wrist inward toward body so that pole is extending backward over dominant shoulder.
13. Quickly extend elbow upward and forward, simultaneously flexing wrist forward, casting line 1 foot into water.
14. Cast baited fishing line 2 feet into water.

15. Cast baited fishing line 3 feet into water.
16. Cast baited fishing line 4 feet into water.
17. Cast baited fishing line 5 feet into water.

Activity Guidelines/Special Adaptations:
1. The casting motion should be practiced at first with any stick or a yardstick. These will be lighter and easier to manipulate.
2. Handle of fishing rod can be built up with foam padding and tape.
3. A light stick or head pointer can be used with a participant having minimal use of arms and hands. This should only be used when fishing for small fish and participant should be accompanied.
4. Pier fishing can provide relaxation for all individuals. Those in wheelchairs who would like to participate should choose a pier with these qualifications:
   a) access walk to pier from shore must be a minimum of 5 feet wide to allow for turning of wheelchairs
   b) handrails must be provided around the entire pier and, according to the Virginia Commission of Outdoor Recreation, must be 36 inches high and have a 30° angle sloping top for arm and pole rest
   c) a kick plate must be provided to prevent foot pedals of wheelchairs from going off the pier
   d) a smooth, nonslip surface must be provided on the access walk and on the pier

Name of Activity: Catch A Fish

Instructional Objective: Given a baited hook in the water, the participant will wait appropriately for the fish to bite and reel it in, 80% of the time.

Materials: baited fishhook, fishing rod and line (with bobber attached)

Verbal Cue: "Kathy, watch the bobber."

Task Analysis:
1. Cast baited fishing line into water.
2. Keeping silent and standing still, focus on bobber floating on surface of water.
3. When bobber disappears beneath the surface, a fish is on the hook.
4. Quickly bend elbow of dominant arm upward, jerking line and fish out of water.
5. Keeping fish out of water, walk away from water.
6. Extend elbow downward, lowering fish onto ground.
7. Bend knees, lowering body toward ground.
8. Extend fingers of dominant hand, releasing pole onto ground.

Activity Guidelines/Special Adaptations:
1. An excellent way to discover when a fish is biting or caught on the hook is to attach a bobber (float) to the line that will float on the water's surface. When a fish bites the hook it is pulled below the surface.
2. An area where most participants will get the opportunity to fish is along the shore. Areas along bodies of water that provide for fishing must have the following standards to facilitate disabled persons:
    a) fishing area must have a level, hard-surfaced area extending 8 feet from the shore, accessible by walks
    b) a handrail must be placed along the shoreline
    c) benches must be provided in the fishing area along the bank
3. Pulling in a fish may be made into a cooperative skill requiring the teamwork of at least two individuals. As one pulls the fish in, the other may stand nearby with a net in hand. As the fish is raised out of the water, the other person positions the net (open and facing upward) underneath the fish, catching the fish in the net.
4. Another person may also hold onto the fisherman's waist to keep him from falling over when attempting to pull in the fish.
5. No one should ever fish alone. A supervisor (that is, an established swimmer with an updated senior lifesaving certificate) must accompany those fishing at all times.

HANDBALL

Name of Activity: Put On Glove

Instructional Objective: Given a handball glove, the participant will put the glove on his dominant hand, 100% of the time.
Materials: handball glove
Verbal Cue: "Paul, put the glove on."

Task Analysis:
1. Extend nondominant arm downward toward glove, palm face down, thumb and index finger extended.
2. Lower nondominant arm until thumb and index finger make contact with opposite sides of open end of glove.
3. Apply inward pressure between thumb and index finger to grasp glove firmly.
4. Bend elbow, raising glove to chest level.
5. Extend dominant arm outward toward opening of glove, palm faced down, fingers extended and spread apart slightly.

6. Position dominant hand directly in front of opening of glove (glove faced downward).
7. Extend elbow of dominant arm, moving hand outward into opening of glove.
8. Continue extending elbow, moving hand into glove with appropriate fingers in fingers of glove, simultaneously bending elbow of nondominant arm, moving hand inward toward body, pulling glove onto dominant hand.

Activity Guidelines/Special Adaptations:
1. Leather gloves should be treated with preservatives and softeners or they can lose their flexibility and become difficult to put on. Gloves with velcro fasteners may be preferable to those with conventional snaps for persons with impaired fine motor dexterity.
2. A larger glove can be worn in order to make it easier to slide the hand and fingers into the glove.

Name of Activity: Serve Handball

Instructional Objective: Given a handball and a handball glove, the participant will serve the handball, hitting it at least 5 feet, 80% of the time.

Materials: handball, handball glove

Verbal Cue: "Paul, serve the ball."

Task Analysis:
1. Bounce ball.
2. As ball ascends, position palm of dominant hand directly behind ball.
3. Quickly extend elbow, moving hand outward away from body against ball, hitting ball forward 1 foot.
4. Hit ball 2 feet.
5. Hit ball 3 feet.
6. Hit ball 4 feet.
7. Hit ball 5 feet against wall, serving ball.

Activity Guidelines/Special Adaptations:
1. A tee similar to that used for holding a baseball stationary may be used if participant has excessive difficulty coordinating movement of both hands.
2. If participant has use of only one hand, he can toss the ball and serve it with the same hand.
3. A leadup activity to serving is bouncing the ball and catching it in the air.

4. Participant should keep his eyes on the ball while serving.
5. Serving arm should be fully extended with the hand perpendicular to floor.
6. A larger ball (e.g., beach ball) can be used to help participant with impaired eye-hand coordination. With proficiency, however, smaller balls should be used.

Name of Activity: Hit Ball Against Wall

Instructional Objective: Given a handball and a handball glove, the participant will hit the ball that is bouncing toward him with dominant hand a distance of 5 feet, 80% of the time.
Materials: handball, handball glove
Verbal Cue: "Paul, hit the ball."

Task Analysis:
1. Serve ball against wall.
2. As ball rebounds and bounces off floor, run toward ball with dominant hand positioned directly behind ball.
3. When ball is within arm's reach, move gloved hand forward toward ball until contact is made with ball.
4. Continue moving hand forward against ball, hitting ball forward 1 foot.
5. Hit ball 2 feet.
6. Hit ball 3 feet.
7. Hit ball 4 feet.
8. Hit ball 5 feet.

Activity Guidelines/Special Adaptations:
1. This can best be practiced against a wall in an enclosed area to minimize the amount of time spent chasing the ball.
2. Initially, bounce ball toward participant with a high bounce that is nearly perpendicular to ground. This will give him ample time to strike the ball. This skill can also be practiced using a stationary ball suspended from a string at midchest level.
3. The game of tetherball is an enjoyable means of improving handball skills. Hitting the attached ball around a pole requires the same motion as hitting a handball.

JOGGING

Name of Activity: Arm-Leg Rotation

Instructional Objective: Given a line 5 feet away, the participant will run to the line, displaying proper arm-leg rotation, 80% of the time.

Materials: running shoes, floor marker
Verbal Cue: "Kate, run to the line."

Task Analysis:
1. Stand with feet on ground, shoulder-width apart.
2. Bend arms at elbows, bringing elbows to waist level, arms facing forward and perpendicular to body.
3. Lift right foot 6 inches off ground by raising knee.
4. Extend right leg forward.
5. At same time right foot is raised, extend left arm in forward direction.
6. Place heel of right foot on ground.
7. Lift left foot 6 inches off ground by raising knee.
8. Extend left leg forward.
9. At same time left foot is raised, bring left arm back to bent 90° angle position and extend right arm in forward direction.
10. Place heel of left foot on ground.
11. Jog 2 feet displaying arm-leg rotation.
12. Jog 3 feet.
13. Jog 4 feet.
14. Jog 5 feet.

Activity Guidelines/Special Adaptations:
1. The proper jogging arm-leg rotation can be taught using a matching cadence.
2. The alternate arm-leg rotation is easily observed when viewing a film (preferably in slow motion) of an Olympic runner. Special Olympics has an excellent film and slide presentation depicting the components of the smooth integrated run (or jog).

PLAYGROUND EQUIPMENT

Name of Activity: See-Saw Play

Instructional Objective: Given an 8-foot see-saw, the participant will raise and lower the see-saw while sitting on it with another player, 3 consecutive times, 80% of the time.
Materials: see-saw
Verbal Cue: "Lisa, ride the see-saw."

Task Analysis:
1. Stand facing left side of see-saw, feet parallel and 6 inches apart.
2. Bend knee of right leg, lifting foot over seat of see-saw.
3. Lower body to see-saw.

4. Lower right foot to ground.
5. Extend arms outward toward handles of see-saw, palms faced down.
6. Lower arms until palms make contact with handles.
7. Curl fingers around handle.
8. Wrap thumbs around opposite side of handle.
9. Apply inward pressure between thumbs and fingers to grasp handle firmly.
10. Extend knees, pushing off with feet, raising see-saw into air.
11. As see-saw descends, lower feet onto ground, bending knees as see-saw touches ground.
12. Go up and down on see-saw second time.
13. Go up and down on see-saw third time.

Activity Guidelines/Special Adaptations:
1. If it is believed that the participant cannot hold onto the handle and remain seated when lifted into the air on the see-saw, the teacher may initially sit on the see-saw behind the participant. In this way, the danger of participant falling off is diminished and the range of motion is still experienced.
2. Before a conventional playground see-saw is used, a miniature one should be practiced on. A Gym-Dandy Space Rocker works the same way except that the participants are not raised into the air and the danger of falling to the ground is reduced. This Space Rocker seats 3 persons (1 in the center) and is an excellent means for participants to learn appropriate see-saw body movements.

Name of Activity: Sliding Board Play

Instructional Objective: Given an 8-foot sliding board, the participant will climb up the ladder and slide down the board to the ground, 80% of the time.

Materials: 8-foot sliding board

Verbal Cue: "Lisa, climb up the sliding board and go down."

Task Analysis:
1. Stand directly in front of the ladder, feet parallel and 6 inches apart.
2. Extend both arms outward toward rungs of ladder, palms faced down.
3. Lower arms until palms make contact with rungs.
4. Curl fingers around rungs.
5. Wrap thumbs around opposite sides of rungs.
6. Apply inward pressure between thumbs and fingers to grasp rungs firmly.

7. Bend knee of dominant leg, raising foot to first step.
8. Lower dominant foot to first step.
9. Bend knee of nondominant leg, raising foot to first step.
10. Lower nondominant foot to first step.
11. Climb rest of steps to top of slide, sliding hands upward on rungs to maintain balance while climbing.
12. Bend knee of dominant leg, lifting foot over top of ladder.
13. Extend knee fully, placing leg onto sliding board.
14. Bend knee of nondominant leg, lifting foot over top of ladder.
15. Extend knee fully, placing leg onto sliding board, assuming a sitting position.
16. Lean forward at waist.
17. Lower arms to sliding board, palms faced down.
18. Extend elbows, pushing off from board with hands, pushing body down slide.
19. When participant reaches bottom, lower feet onto ground to stop momentum.
20. Extend knees, raising body to upright position.

Activity Guidelines/Special Adaptations:
1. A soft, sandy, or padded area should be located directly beneath the bottom of the slide. This activity becomes enjoyable when the participants are aware that they will be landing on a soft area. A pile of pillows may also be used for this purpose.
2. If it is felt that participant may have difficulty climbing the ladder, the teacher should stand on the ladder directly behind the participant so that there is no danger of participant falling off the ladder while climbing. Also, a smaller portable sliding board may be used. An apparatus of this nature may be safer because it has only 1 or 2 steps to climb before getting to the top.
3. A wider slide may be used, making it less likely for a participant to fall off while descending. Additionally, the sides of the sliding board can be built up, making it nearly impossible for any participant to fall off the side of the board before sliding to the bottom. Waxed paper can be placed under participant, making it easier to slide down the board.
4. Slides for disabled individuals must provide access to all types of handicaps. To meet this demand, the following criteria should be met:
   a) No ladders and legs can be used on slides
   b) Slides must be embedded in a mound
   c) Access to the top of the slide must be via a ramp or series of ramps

d) Grab bars must be provided along ramps and top and bottom of slide to accommodate semiambulant participants

Name of Activity: Swing Play

Instructional Objective: Given a swing set, the participant will sit on the swing and swing 5 feet forward and 5 feet backward without stopping, 80% of the time.

Materials: swing set

Verbal Cue: "Lisa, swing back and forth."

Task Analysis:
1. Stand with feet parallel and 6 inches apart, with swing directly behind backside.
2. Bend knees, lowering body until calves form 90° angle to thighs and buttocks make contact with seat of swing.
3. Extend knees, pushing body completely onto swing seat.
4. Extend both arms upward toward chains, palms faced inward on outer side of chains.
5. Curl fingers around outer side of chains.
6. Wrap thumbs around opposite side of chains.
7. Apply inward pressure between thumbs and fingers to grasp chains firmly.
8. Push off ground with balls of feet by extending knees, causing swing to move backward.
9. As swing moves backward, bend knees, moving legs back behind swing, leaning forward slightly at waist.
10. As swing moves forward, lean backward slightly at waist, extending knees, bring legs forward in front of swing.
11. Swing back and forth second time.
12. Swing back and forth third time.
13. Extend knees, lowering feet to ground, dragging feet on ground until swing stops moving.

Activity Guidelines/Special Adaptations:
1. Allow participants to hold on to the chains of the swing in a manner that is most comfortable for them. Overhand, underhand, and mixed grips can be used.
2. Initially, the teacher may push the swing from behind, allowing the participant to experience the swinging motion. This assistance should be faded out until participant is eventually propelling swing on her own.
3. A swing set is available that seats 2 persons at the same time. It

requires the pushing and pulling of a bar with the arms to get the swing in motion. This would be excellent for nonambulatory persons since leg movements are not necessary.
4. Box-type swings can be used that have a safety bar in front that can be held for security and balance, as well as serving to keep participant stationary.

SHUFFLEBOARD

Name of Activity: Line Up Discs

Instructional Objective: Given a regulation shuffleboard set, the participant will line up 4 discs in the appropriate place, 80% of the time.
Materials: regulation shuffleboard set with 4 discs
Verbal Cue: "Dennis, line up the discs."

Task Analysis:
1. Extend dominant arm downward toward first disc, palm faced down, thumb and index finger extended.
2. Lower arm until thumb and index finger make contact with opposite sides of edge of disc.
3. Apply inward pressure between thumb and index finger to grasp disc firmly.
4. Bend elbow, raising disc to waist level.
5. Extend dominant arm holding disc outward to the "10 off" block adjacent to front edge and left of center line.
6. Lower arm until disc makes contact with ground.
7. Extend thumb and index finger, releasing disc onto ground.
8. Pick up second disc.
9. Position second disc adjacent to and left of first disc in "10 off" box.
10. Place second disc on ground.
11. Place third disc adjacent to and left of second disc.
12. Place forth disc adjacent to and left of third disc.

Activity Guidelines/Special Adaptations:
1. Center line of playing board can be extended into "10 off" box to aid participant with correct disc placement.
2. 2-by 4-inch pieces of wood can be used to build up front of "10 off" box and facilitate alignment of discs.
3. Outlines of 8 discs can be drawn on playing board at starting line. Each participant would be required to position his 4 discs inside the outlines.

Sports   149

Name of Activity: Shoot Disc

Instructional Objective: Given a regulation shuffleboard set, the participant will shoot a disc 5 feet toward the target area, 80% of the time.
Materials: regulation shuffleboard set
Verbal Cue: "Dennis, shoot a disc."

Task Analysis:
1. Line up disc along edge of starting line, opposite from and 5 feet away from target area.
2. Hold shuffleboard stick.
3. Position open end of head of stick directly against back of disc (participant is standing facing target area).
4. Lean forward slightly at waist.
5. Extend elbow of dominant arm, moving arm forward, pushing stick against disc, propelling disc forward 1 foot.
6. Shoot disc 2 feet.
7. Shoot disc 3 feet.
8. Shoot disc 4 feet.
9. Shoot disc 5 feet to target area.

Activity Guidelines/Special Adaptations:
1. In some cases, it may be advisable to increase or decrease the distance from starting line to scoring box, depending upon the ability and strength of the individual.
2. Target area may be the actual shuffleboard court, a large circle, or any other designated area that makes it easier to score points.
3. Boundaries (walls) made of wood may be positioned on each side of the target area to assure an accurate shot. This will increase self-esteem and also prevent the discs from leaving the playing area.

SOFTBALL

Name of Activity: Underhand Throw

Instructional Objective: Given a softball, the participant will throw the ball underhand a distance of 5 feet, 80% of the time.
Materials: softball
Verbal Cue: "Amos, throw the ball underhand."

Task Analysis:
1. Stand directly behind softball, feet parallel and 6 inches apart.
2. Bend knees, lowering body toward ground.
3. Extend dominant arm outward toward ball, palm faced down.

4. Lower dominant arm until palm makes contact with ball.
5. Curl fingers around ball.
6. Wrap thumb around opposite side of ball.
7. Apply inward pressure between thumb and fingers to grasp ball firmly.
8. Bend elbow, bringing ball to waist level.
9. Straighten knees, raising body to upright position.
10. Extend elbow, bringing arm outward to dominant side of body.
11. Extend elbow, moving arm backward behind body, forming a 45° angle with back of body.
12. Rotate wrist so that palm of hand is facing forward.
13. Extend elbow, swinging arm forward to front of body in a pendulum motion, simultaneously shifting weight to dominant foot.
14. When elbow is fully extended outward, extend fingers, releasing ball in forward direction 1 foot.
15. Throw ball 2 feet.
16. Throw ball 3 feet.
17. Throw ball 4 feet.
18. Throw ball 5 feet.

Activity Guidelines/Special Adaptations:
1. This skill may initially be taught using a foam rubber Nerf ball that is the same size as a softball. This will allow instruction for persons having difficulty grasping and who lack the necessary strength to pick up a softball.
2. The underhand throwing motion may be practiced by swinging the throwing arm back and forth by the side of the body. The teacher can also explain to the participant that this is same underhand motion as used in bowling.

Name of Activity; Catch Ball

Instructional Objective: Given a mitt and a softball, the participant will catch the ball thrown from a distance of 6 feet, 80% of the time.
Materials: softball, mitt
Verbal Cue: "Amos, catch the ball."

Task Analysis:
1. Place mitt on nondominant hand.
2. Bend mitted arm at elbow, forming a 90° angle with body, forearm parallel to ground.
3. Rotate wrist so that palm of mitted hand is facing upward.
4. Open mitt by extending fingers.
5. Follow flight of ball through air.

6. Position palm of mitt directly in path of approaching ball.
7. When ball makes contact with mitt, move dominant arm sideways at shoulder, bringing arm toward ball.
8. Bend elbow of dominant arm until palm of dominant arm makes contact with ball in mitt.
9. Bend elbow, moving arms inward to chest, catching ball.

Activity Guidelines/Special Adaptations:
1. A beanbag may be used instead of a softball in order to make catching easier. The softer the object thrown, the easier it will be to catch and hold it; this will also alleviate a participant's fear of being hit by a thrown object. A harder ball has a tendency to bounce out of mitt or hand, whereas a beanbag or similar object will land and remain in mitt.
2. A balloon is an exceptionally good object to use when first learning to catch because it travels slowly through the air.
3. Have the participant catch a ball that is thrown from 1 foot away. With proficiency, increase the distance until criterion is met.
4. Initially, participants can learn to catch a ball without the use of a baseball mitt. When proficiency is demonstrated, a mitt may be introduced into the skill.

Name of Activity: Hit Ball

Instructional Objective: Given a baseball bat, a softball, and a batting tee, the participant will hit the ball with the bat 10 feet, 80% of the time.

Materials: baseball bat, softball, batting tee

Verbal Cue: "Amos, hit the ball."

Task Analysis:
1. Stand to one side of batting tee so that nondominant shoulder is facing tee with feet parallel and 6 inches apart.
2. Keep eyes focused on ball on batting tee.
3. Swing baseball bat.
4. Extend elbows, bringing bat downward and forward toward ball.
5. Make contact with ball.
6. Follow through with bay by continuing swing until arms are fully extended and locked at nondominant side of body.
7. Make sure eyes are focused on ball at all times.
8. Hit ball 2 feet.
9. Hit ball 4 feet.
10. Hit ball 6 feet.
11. Hit ball 8 feet.
12. Hit ball 10 feet.

Activity Guidelines/Special Adaptations:
1. Batting positions for a left-hander: nondominant shoulder to tee, but must be parallel when it hits the ball, the follow through requires crossing the midline of the body.
2. After the participant has mastered the skill of hitting the ball off the tee, the tee may be removed and the ball can be pitched (underhand throw) to batter.
3. Teacher should remind players to watch the bat hit the ball. There is never a point in the swing when the batter does not have his eyes focused on the ball.
4. Adjustable batting tees are available that can be raised from 27 inches to 43 inches. Any kind of ball can be used with the batting tee.
5. A ball can also be suspended from the ceiling. Using this technique eliminates the need for retrieving balls.

SWIMMING

Name of Activity: Enter Swimming Pool

Instructional Objective: Given a swimming pool with a water depth of 3 feet, the participant will enter the pool and stand in waist high water for 1 minute, 100% of the time.

Materials: swimming pool (3-foot water depth)

Verbal Cue: "Billy, get into the water."

Task analysis:
1. Walk to ladder of swimming pool.
2. Extend dominant arm outward toward ladder railing, palm faced down.
3. Lower arm until palm makes contact with railing.
4. Curl fingers around top of railing.
5. Wrap thumb around opposite side of top of railing.
6. Apply inward pressure to grasp railing firmly.
7. Bend knee of right leg, raising foot 3 inches off step.
8. Lower foot to next step by extending knee.
9. Step down to same step with left foot.
10. Step down to next step with right foot.
11. Step down to same step with left foot.
12. Step down to pool floor with right foot.
13. Step down to pool floor with left foot.
14. Stand in water for 5 seconds.
15. Stand in water for 10 seconds.
16. Stand in water for 15 seconds.

17. Stand in water for 30 seconds.
18. Stand in water for 1 minute.

Activity Guidelines/Special Adaptations:
1. Because of the inherent dangers involved in any swimming program, it is highly recommended that a one-to-one instructional basis be used.
2. A slight elevation around the pool provides safety against accidentally falling in while walking around the deck. A safety precaution that is always helpful is the use of the "buddy system."
3. Steps with handrails leading into the water should be built with short tiers and a wide step to provide for easy entrance and exit. In some cases, rails are fixed across pool to permit participants to hold on and gain a feeling of security.
4. Pool steps should be widely spaced and have smooth with handrails available.
5. Floating cork ropes can be used to divide pool into deep and shallow end and may be used to help find way to ladder.

Name of Activity: Walk Through Water

Instructional Objective: Given a swimming pool with a water depth of 3 feet, the participant will walk 10 feet to the instructor, 100% of the time.

Materials: swimming pool (3-foot water depth)

Verbal Cue: "Billy, come to me."

Task Analysis:
1. Enter swimming pool and adjust to water.
2. Stand by side of pool in shallow end.
3. Place palm of hand closest to wall on gutter of pool.
4. Grasp gutter firmly between fingers and thumb on upper and lower side of gutter.
5. Apply inward finger pressure to grasp gutter firmly.
6. Place one foot in front of the other and take step toward instructor.
7. Continue forward foot placement to walk 1 foot toward instructor.
8. Walk 3 feet toward instructor.
9. Walk 5 feet toward instructor.
10. Walk 10 feet toward instructor.

Activity Guidelines/Special Adaptations:
1. Participant should use some form of flotation device until his ability level is assessed.

2. Rough-textured tile on the bottom of the pool will allow for better traction and will prevent slipping.
3. There should be an area in the pool with handrails for practice. The participant can hold the rail while walking to the instructor. The comfort of grasping the instructor's hand may be quite reinforcing, too.
4. Practice walking in shallow water (waist deep) and move progressively to deeper water.
5. There should be a fairly large area containing shallow water to permit casual water play for participants lacking the skills required to play in the deeper end.

Name of Activity: Breath Control

Instructional Objective: Given a swimming pool with a water depth of 3 feet, the participant will place his face in the water and hold his breath for 2 seconds, 80% of the time.

Materials: swimming pool (3-foot water depth)

Verbal Cue: "Billy, put your face in the water."

Task Analysis:
1. Enter swimming pool and adjust to water.
2. Bend slightly at knees to lower head toward water.
3. Extend arms downward toward knees.
4. Place palms of hands on knees.
5. Lower head toward water.
6. Take deep breath.
7. Close mouth to retain air—do not exhale.
8. Lower face to water by bending forward at waist.
9. Place mouth on top of water.
10. Part lips slightly.
11. Blow bubbles through mouth.
12. Raise head from water.
13. Take deep breath.
14. Lower face to water.
15. Place mouth, nose, and eyes in water.
16. Part lips slightly.
17. Blow air out through mouth to exhale.
18. Raise head.
19. Take deep breath.
20. Lower face into water until water level is up to ears.
21. Keep mouth and nose under water for 1 second, holding breath.

22. Hold breath under water for 2 seconds.
23. Raise head from water.
24. Take deep breath.

Activity Guidelines/Special Adapatations:
1. Participants must initially learn to hold their breath out of the swimming pool before attempting to hold breath in the water.
2. Prior to getting into the pool, the task can be done in a pan of water, in order to get participant conditioned.
3. Have swimmer sit on teacher's lap in water and on count of 3, teacher bends knees and both go under water together. This gives the participant a feeling of security.
4. Use ping pong balls to teach participants to exhale through mouth, then nose, to move ball through water. This activity can initially get participant's face near the water.
5. Blowing games can be played in or out of the water; they are important leadup activities to rhythmic breathing. Have participants blow a ping pong ball, toy boat, or sponge across the pool.

VOLLEYBALL

Name of Activity: Underhand Serve

Instructional Objective: Given a volleyball and a net, the participant will serve the ball over the net in an underhand fashion from 10 feet away, 80% of the time.

Materials: volleyball, net

Verbal Cue: "Jessica, serve the ball."

Task Analysis:
1. Stand directly behind ball, feet parallel and 6 inches apart.
2. Bend knees, lowering body toward ground.
3. Extend arms outward toward opposite sides of ball, palms faced inward.
4. Move arms inward at shoulders until palms make contact with sides of ball.
5. Apply inward pressure between hands to grasp ball firmly.
6. Bend elbows, bringing ball to chest.
7. Extend knees, raising body to upright position.
8. Walk to back right corner of court behind end line and stand facing net 10 feet away.
9. Rotate both wrists counterclockwise so that dominant hand is resting on top of ball and nondominanat hand is supporting ball on the bottom.

10. Extend fingers of dominant hand releasing ball onto palm of nondominant hand.
11. Extend elbow of nondominant arm, moving ball outward to front of body.
12. Curl fingers of dominant hand inward to palm, making a fist.
13. Extend elbow of dominant arm, bringing fist downward to side of body.
14. Quickly bend elbow, raising fist upward and outward to lower half of ball.
15. Extend elbow, continuing to raise fist upward against ball, hitting it forward, serving ball 2 feet.
16. Serve ball 4 feet.
17. Serve ball 6 feet.
18. Serve ball 8 feet.
19. Serve ball 10 feet over net.

Activity Guidelines/Special Adaptations:
1. The underhand serve may be performed with a closed fisted hand or with an open hand (hitting ball with heel of palm). The ball will usually travel further when a fist is used.
2. Initially, the participant should serve the ball a short distance from the net to assure success. As players progress, continue moving them further back until they are serving from the end line (right corner).
3. To improve eye-hand coordination and make the task easier, the participant can practice the serving motion with a ballon instead of the standard volleyball. The balloon may not be hit over the net, but it is a good way to practice the proper underhand motion. Also, the balloon is easier to hold in the nondominant hand while hitting with the other hand.

Name of Activity: Return Ball Over Net

Instructional Objective: Given a net and a volleyball that has been hit toward participant, the participant will hit the ball over the net from 5 feet away, 80% of the time.
Materials: volleyball, net
Verbal Cue: "Jessica, hit the ball over the net."

Task Analysis:
1. Stand 5 feet away from and facing net.
2. Follow flight of ball through air.
3. Extend arms outward toward ball, palms faced down, fingers extended.

4. Bend elbows, bringing hands to head level, simultaneously rotating wrists backward so that palms are faced up.
5. As ball descends, position palms directly below ball.
6. Extend arms upward toward ball until palms make contact with ball, simultaneously extending at knees, applying upward and forward pressure onto ball with hands, hitting ball 1 foot.
7. Hit ball 2 feet.
8. Hit ball 3 feet.
9. Hit ball 4 feet.
10. Hit ball 5 feet, returning ball over net.

Activity Guidelines/Special Adaptations:
1. An excellent leadup skill to volleyball is newcomb. In this game, instead of being required to return the ball over the net, the players only have to catch it and then throw the ball back over the net to the other team. When this game is mastered, the participants will be ready to learn to return a ball by hitting it over the net.
2. A balloon can be used instead of a volleyball to practice hitting over the net. The balloon will significantly slow down the pace of the game. Additionally, the balloon is lighter and the participants will quickly find out that it is much easier to hit the balloon up and over the net than to hit the volleyball.
3. Another way to slow down the pace of the game is to release some air from the volleyball, making it softer.

WEIGHTLIFTING

Name of Activity: Curl

Instructional Objective: Given a 6-lb. dumbbell, the participant will complete one curl, 80% of the time.
Materials: 6-lb. dumbbell
Verbal Cue: "Lucas, do a curl."

Task Analysis:
1. Lift dumbbell to dominant side of body.
2. Raise dominant hand upward toward chest by bending at elbow, with dumbbell in hand.
3. Keep back straight.
4. Continue to bend elbow to raise dumbbell to chest.
5. Slowly lower weight back to side (starting position) by extending arm downward.

Activity Guidelines/Special Adaptations:
1. Curling motion without a dumbbell should be practiced before the participant attempts to complete a curl with the dumbbell.
2. A proper curl is performed with the use of the arm only. Emphasize to participant that the back should be kept erect and that he should use only the elbow and lower arm to lift dumbbell.
3. Arm curl should be performed with each arm individually, to ensure equal muscle development in both arms.

Name of Activity: Lift Weight Over Head

Instructional Objective: Given a 6-lb. dumbbell, the participant will complete one overhead lift, 80% of the time.
Materials: 6-lb. dumbbell
Verbal Cue: "Lucas, lift the dumbbell over your head."

Task Analysis:
1. Complete a curl with dominant arm, bringing dumbbell to chest.
2. Rotate wrist until length of dumbbell is parallel to side of body.
3. Extend arm straight upward and overhead by extending elbow.
4. Lower arm and dumbbell to neck height by bending at elbow.
5. Slowly lower forearm to side of body by extending elbow until dumbbell is at waist level and not more than 6 inches from side of body.

Activity Guidelines/Special Adaptations:
1. The overhead lifting motion without a dumbbell should be practiced before participant attempts to complete an overhead lift with the dumbbell.
2. Overhead lift should be performed with each arm individually, so as to ensure equal muscle development in both arms.

WINTER SPORTS

Name of Activity: Make Snowball

Instructional Objective: Given a handful of snow, the participant will shape it into a snowball at least 2 inches in diameter, 80% of the time.
Materials: handful of snow.
Verbal Cue: "Sonya, make a snowball."

Task Analysis:
1. Put on gloves.
2. Extend dominant arm downward toward snow, palm faced inward.

3. Bring four fingers of dominant hand together until there are no spaces between fingers.
4. Keep thumb of dominant hand 2 inches apart from other fingers.
5. Place pinky side of dominant hand into snow by extending arm at elbow.
6. Bend fingers 2 inches to cup hand.
7. Move dominant hand forward toward body 4 inches, scooping snow in process.
8. Close dominant hand around snow.
9. Rotate wrist until palm is facing upward, snow resting on palm.
10. Lift dominant hand with snow in it by bending at elbow.
11. Bring four fingers of nondominant hand together until there are no spaces between fingers.
12. Keep thumb of nondominant hand 2 inches apart from other fingers.
13. Bend fingers of nondominant hand 2 inches to cup hand.
14. Place palm of nondominant hand on top of snow in dominant hand.
15. Raise nondominant hand from snow 1 inch by raising lower arm at elbow.
16. Lower nondominant hand to snow.
17. Raise and lower nondominant hand until ball shape is formed.
18. Pack snow by pressing palms of hands together from either side until a snowball, 2 inches in diameter, is formed.

Activity Guidelines/Special Adaptations:
1. A one pint plastic container may be used to scoop the snow if participant is unable to do so with hands.
2. Smaller snowballs can be made using a spring-operated ice cream scoop.
3. Snow is easier to pack and make into a snowball if it is wet, not powdery. Increase the opportunity for success by using snow that is easily packed.

Name of Activity: Sledding

Instructional Objective: Given a sled 4 feet long, the participant will coast straight down a hill 6 feet without falling off, 80% of the time.
Materials: sled (4 feet long), hill with snow
Verbal Cue: "Sonya, sled down the hill."

Task Analysis:
1. Stand facing sled with feet parallel, shoulder width apart.
2. Raise left foot off ground by raising knee.
3. Place left foot to left side of sled, 4 inches away from sled.
4. Raise right foot off ground by raising knee.

5. Place right foot on right side of sled, 4 inches away from sled.
6. Lower body to sled, 1½ feet from front of sled, by bending at knees to sitting position.
7. Place palms of hands on either side of sled, 1 foot behind heels of feet.
8. Apply inward finger pressure to grasp both sides of sled firmly.
9. Push sled backward with both feet by extending at knees, then forward by bending knees toward body.
10. As descent begins, raise feet off ground, placing them on top and 6 inches from front of sled.
11. Keep hands firmly held on sides of sled to balance body and prevent falling off.
12. Travel 1 foot down incline on sled.
13. Travel 3 feet down hill on sled.
14. Travel 6 feet down hill on sled to bottom of hill.

Activity Guidelines/Special Adaptations:
1. Sled runners should be free of rust and rubbed with paraffin or waxed paper to allow sled to move easily through snow.
2. Choose a hill with sufficient incline to allow participant a good ride without unnecessary risk of losing control of sled.
3. If sled is long enough, two people can ride down hill together. This may be necessary to initially give participant confidence to sled independently.
4. If sled runners present too great a risk, a toboggan that has a flat bottom, or a sledding disc can be used.

Chapter 8
GAMES

One may question the function and value of a game. Games (e.g., board and table, motor, musical, cards) can provide opportunities for cooperation, success, learning to accept failure gracefully, taking turns, adhering to roles, sharing, and enjoyment. Unlike unrestricted toy play, all games contain certain rules and procedures that must be followed. They can be highly organized with a specific goal, or less systematic, open-ended, and flexible to permit a minimum of competition. In the latter, participation is for the mere sake of obtaining pleasure within a recreative experience. Games calling for minimal competition can be introduced to children and used with more rigid rules and goals by more capable persons. Modifications of game rules and materials are endless, enhancing participation of the lower functioning individual. Several games in this chapter require special materials (e.g., game board, moving pieces); others require nothing but the participants themselves.

The 33 games in this chapter include:

Age Level*	Games	Page
	BOARD AND TABLE GAMES	
C/A	Bingo	162
C/A	Checkers	163
C/A	Crossword Puzzle	164
C/A	Darts	165
C	Jacks	166
C	Lotto	167
C	Marbles	168
C/A	Pinball	169
C/A	Ping Pong	170
C/A	Tic-tac-toe	171
	MOTOR GAMES	
C/A	Arm Wrestle	172
C	Follow the Leader	173
C/A	Hand Slap	174
C	Hopscotch	175
C/A	Jump Rope	176
C	Kickball	177
C	Parachute Play	178
C	Simon Says	179
C	Tag	180
C/A	Tetherball	181
C/A	Tug of War	183
C/A	Twister	183

* C, Indicates chronologically age-appropriate for child; A, Indicates chronologically age-appropriate for adolescent and adult; C/A, Indicates chronologically age-appropriate for child, adolescent, and adult.

161

MUSICAL/RHYTHMICAL GAMES

C	Farmer in the Dell	184
C/A	Home Rhythm Band	185
C	Hot Potato	186
C/A	Limbo	187
C	London Bridge	188
C/A	Musical Chairs	189

CARD GAMES

C/A	Concentration	190
C/A	I Doubt It	191
C/A	Old Maid	192
C/A	Slap Jack	193
C/A	War	194

BOARD AND TABLE GAMES

Name of Activity: Bingo

Instructional Objective: Given a 5 by 5 square bingo board and 25 flat circular markers, the participant will place a marker on each square called by the caller until he has 5 marked squares in a row, horizontally, vertically, or diagonally, and calls "bingo," 80% of the time.

Materials: bingo board (5 by 5 square), circular markers, caller

Verbal Cue: "Herman, play bingo."

Task Analysis:
1. Extend dominant hand toward marker.
2. Grasp marker using pincer grasp.
3. Attend to call made by caller.
4. Locate square called by caller.
5. Extend dominant hand toward bingo board.
6. Lower dominant hand until marker touches square.
7. Release marker onto square by extending fingers.
8. Continue playing game until 5 squares in a row have been marked.
9. Call "bingo."

Activity Guidelines/Special Adaptations:
1. A 3 by 3 square board (limited range and amount of matches) will be easier to use for lower functioning players. Each square should have one number, letter, picture, color, or shape in it. Letters across top of card can be omitted.
2. Bingo cards, secured to table with masking tape, and built-in sliding markers are helpful for motor impaired players. Cards and chips can also be made larger for easier manipulation.
3. Caller can bring card containing number, letter, or picture next to the

board of any player having difficulty finding match. Picture should always be held up concurrently with each call.
4. Any matching activities (worksheets, cards, lotto) are good leadup activities for bingo.
5. Bingo is a practical activity for large groups. Prizes may be awarded to winners.
6. An adaptation for visually impaired persons can be made by providing board with raised numerals or letters or braille symbols.
7. "Pop-O-Matic" bingo game is commercially available. This game enables many physically handicapped participants to be callers because the pop-o-matic dome can be pushed with any part of body.
8. During a holiday season (e.g., Halloween) the game can be played using pictures appropriate to specific season (e.g., witch, moon, candy corn) on playing cards.
9. Lines between boxes on playing cards can be built up with cardboard requiring participant to drop chip into boxed-in square.

Name of Activity: Checkers

Instructional Objective: Given a checkerboard with playing discs in standard formation, the participant will move discs in a diagonal pattern toward the opponent's side of the board, jumping qualified playing discs belonging to the opponent, 80% of the time.

Materials: 24 checkers, checkerboard

Verbal Cue: "Roselyn, play checkers."

Task Analysis:
1. Extend dominant hand downward toward board and playing discs.
2. Visually locate one appropriate disc for move.
3. Grasp disc with pincer grasp.
4. Slide disc to nearest open diagonal space, by extending dominant arm outward away from body.
5. Wait for opponent to take his turn.
6. Continue playing until opponent's disc is in position to be jumped.

To Jump A Disc:
7. Extend dominant hand downward toward disc to be moved.
8. Grasp disc using pincer grasp.
9. Raise arm lifting disc 2 inches off checkerboard.
10. Move disc diagonally over opponent's disc to next available free space.
11. Release grasp on disc by extending fingers.
12. Extend dominant hand to opponent's jumped disc.

13. Grasp disc using pincer grasp.
14. Raise disc 2 inches off checkerboard.
15. Extend dominant hand to dominant side of body, away from checkerboard.
16. Lower dominant hand toward table top.
17. Release grasp on disc to table.
18. Continue playing game until first player has lost all discs.

Activity Guidelines/Special Adaptations:
1. Larger checkerboards can be purchased or made from heavy cardboard or wood.
2. Checkers is a relaxing and quiet game for adult players with physical disabilities.
3. Large nails can be driven into each checker to provide an easier method of moving and manipulating pieces.
4. Discs can also be coded with letter, number, or picture to simplify disc identification process.
5. Discs reaching opponent's home base are crowned kings. At that time, "King me" should be called.
6. The game of "Loser" can be used as an adaptation of checkers. Player who wins, loses game and loser wins. Game is played like checkers except each player tries to lose her discs.

Name of Activity: Crossword Puzzle

Instructional Objective: Given a simple crossword puzzle and pencil, the participant will read description/definition and write word in appropriate numbered box, 25% of the time.

Materials: crossword puzzle, pencil

Verbal Cue: "Charles, do the crossword puzzle."

Task Analysis:
1. Extend dominant arm toward pencil.
2. Grasp pencil using appropriate writing grasp.
3. Extend dominant arm toward crossword puzzle.
4. Read first clue "across."
5. Think of word.
6. Extend dominant hand to 1 "across" box.
7. Write letters or word in appropriate boxes.
8. Read clue 1 "down."
9. Think of word.
10. Extend dominant hand to 1 "down" box.
11. Write letters of word in appropriate boxes.

12. Continue reading clues and filling boxes with appropriate words until puzzle is completed, alternating "across" then "down."

Activity Guidelines/Special Adaptations:
1. In classroom, crossword puzzle can be drawn on blackboard and worked on as group effort.
2. A crossword puzzle is a good independent activity for a student when he finishes another activity before the remainder of his classmates. Encourage participant to work out as much of the puzzle as possible before asking for assistance.
3. When puzzles are worked on independently, answers can be provided on a separate list to reinforce participant immediately.
4. Tape puzzle page on table to aid motor impaired individual with writing answers.
5. Correct answers should be simple; use several two- and three- letter words initially. Illustrations of objects can be given as clues so that participant only needs to spell word.
6. Puzzles can be used as class lessons, using clues such as parts of body or sounds that animals make.

Name of Activity: Darts

Instructional Objective: Given a dartboard 8 feet away and 3 darts, the participant will throw the darts striking the board, 67% of the time.
Materials: dartboard and 3 darts
Verbal Cue: "Stuart, throw the darts."

Task Analysis:
1. Stand/sit 8 feet from dartboard.
2. Extend dominant hand toward large end of dart.
3. Grasp dart in throwing position using pincer grasp.
4. Bend elbow of dominant arm until forearm is perpendicular to ground in front of body.
5. Thrust arm in forward motion toward dart board by extending elbow, hitting dartboard.
6. Throw second dart, striking dartboard.
7. Throw third dart, striking dartboard.

Activity Guidelines/Special Adaptations:
1. A velcro dartboard or large rubber suction dart game can be used instead of standard dartboard for younger and lower functioning participants.
2. An enlarged dartboard with fewer and larger spaces can be used with darts made larger by wrapping gripping surface.

3. Overhead beanbag tossing activity can be implemented as leadup for player having difficulty manipulating smaller and lighter darts.
4. "Pitch-a-Peg" ring toss game with bull's-eye boards are commercially available or can be made quite simply.
5. "Soft Touch" dart sets with nonmetal flexible dart tips are commercially available. This game looks and plays like a regular dart game, but is much safer.
6. For participants in need of practice, allow them to throw more than 3 darts consecutively at board to get better feel for game and to warm up adequately.
7. Initially, dart throwers can stand 4 feet from dartboard, and with proficiency, increase throwing distance to 5 feet, 6 feet, 7 feet, and ultimately, to regulation distance, 8 feet.

Name of Activity: Jacks

Instructional Objective: Given a set of jacks and a ball, the participant will scatter the jacks, bounce the ball with one hand, pick up a jack with the same hand while the ball is in the air, and then catch the ball with the same hand before it hits the gound, 50% of the time.

Materials: set of 5 standard size jacks, rubber ball (1-inch diameter)

Verbal Cue: "Jay, play jacks."

Task Analysis:
1. Extend dominant arm downward toward 5 jacks.
2. Grasp 5 jacks in dominant hand using palmar grasp.
3. Raise dominant hand 6 inches above ground by bending at elbow.
4. Rotate wrist until palm is facing downward.
5. Extend fingers releasing jacks to ground.
6. Extend dominant hand toward ball.
7. Grasp ball in dominant hand using palmar grasp.
8. Raise dominant hand 6 inches above ground by bending at elbow.
9. Rotate wrist until palm is facing downward.
10. Extend fingers to bounce ball on ground.
11. Quickly drop dominant hand over 1 jack.
12. Grasp jack in dominant hand using palmar grasp.
13. Rotate wrist until palm is facing upward.
14. Place palm underneath ball in flight.
15. Extend fingers of dominant hand until hand is in cupped position.
16. Catch ball in dominant hand using palmar grasp.
17. Release ball onto ground by extending fingers.
18. Grasp remaining jacks using palmar grasp with dominant hand.
19. Raise dominant hand 6 inches above ground.

20. Rotate wrist until palm is facing downward.
21. Release grasp allowing jacks to fall onto ground.
22. Extend dominant hand toward ball.
23. Grasp ball using palmar grasp.
24. Raise hand 6 inches above ground, close to 2 jacks.
25. Rotate wrist until palm is facing upward.
26. Extend fingers, rasing hand upward, releasing ball into air.
27. Quickly drop hand downward over 2 jacks.
28. Grasp 2 jacks with dominant hand using palmar grasp.
29. Rotate wrist until palm is facing upward.
30. Place palm underneath ball in flight.
31. Extend fingers until hand is in cupped position.
32. Catch ball in dominant hand using palmar grasp.
33. Continue game until participant picks up all 5 jacks and catches ball.

Activity Guidelines/Special Adaptations:
1. If it is too difficult to hold previously caught jacks while simultaneously picking up additional ones, jacks can be put aside after they have been picked up.
2. If it is too difficult to catch ball with jacks in hand, jack can be picked up with nondominant hand and ball caught with dominant hand.
3. Game of elevens can be played as simple version of jacks. This game requires participant to place jack in left hand; ball is allowed to bounce before it is caught.
4. Small pebbles can be used instead of jacks, if jacks are unavailable.
5. As opposed to throwing ball and picking up jacks from ground, participant can hold all jacks in hand and place one on ground after ball is thrown and before it is caught. Game ends when all jacks have been put down.

Name of Activity: Lotto

Instructional Objective: Given a Picture Lotto game, the participant will match 5 picture cards correctly to those on his game board, 80% of the time.

Materials: Picture Lotto game

Verbal Cue: "Robert, play Picture Lotto."

Task Analysis:
1. Extend dominant hand downward toward stack of cards.
2. Grasp top card using pincer grasp.
3. Rotate wrist until face of card is in view.
4. Identify picture on card.

5. Match picture to appropriate picture on game board.
6. Release first card onto space by extending fingers.
7. Match second card to game board space.
8. Match third card to game board space.
9. Match fourth card to game board space.
10. Match fifth card to game board space.

Activity Guidelines/Special Adaptations:
1. Shape and Color Lotto can be implemented, depending on participants' needs and ability levels.
2. Begin game using one picture, and with proficiency, include other pictures to be matched.
3. To simplify instruction, those pictures not being used may be covered with paper, leaving only one picture exposed initially. With proficiency, include other pictures of game board and cards.
4. Foam rubber or sand paper (unique textures) can be used for shape lotto if participant has visual impairments.
5. Game can be used as educational experience, and later, to facilitate social interaction in group game.
6. Place picture card to be matched near playing board. Initially, card may be placed adjacent to picture on board to facilitate successful experience.
7. Eventually, use game as bingo game with group; have leader call object names from one spot in room and hold card up for all to see.

Name of Activity: Marbles

Instructional Objective: Given 10 standard size marbles placed in the center of a 12-inch diameter circle and a standard shooter marble, the participant will shoot the shooter marble into the standard marbles knocking at least 1 marble from the circle, 80% of the time.

Materials: 10 standard size marbles, 1 shooter marble, 12-inch diameter circle drawn on the floor.

Verbal Cue: "Miriam, shoot the marble."

Task Analysis:
1. Extend dominant hand downward toward shooter marble.
2. Grasp and hold marble in hollow made by pressing thumb against index finger, 1 inch or 2 inches off ground.
3. Position dominant hand downward toward marbles in circle.
4. Aim shooter marble by placing thumb behind it.
5. Flick thumb forward propelling shooter marble toward other marbles.
6. Knock at least one marble from circle.

Activity Guidelines/Special Adaptations:
1. Larger marbles can ensure greater success for participants.
2. A smaller circle can be used to ensure greater success for participants.
3. Adding a 3-inch high border around a table to keep the marbles from rolling off can make it possible for those players confined to wheelchairs to play the game.
4. A simpler leadup activity can be implemented using beanbags to slide across the floor, knocking other beanbags out of a given circle.
5. After participant becomes proficient with game, a specific number of marbles can be shot out in order to score points.
6. Marbles can also be collected by participant and traded with others to obtain several different colors.
7. A marble game can be played one or two ways. In the first way, the winning score is based on number of marbles hit out of circle. Captured marbles are returned to players at end of game. The second way is to play for keeps, winner captures marbles and keeps them.
8. In most marble games, participants shoot from a predetermined mark (taw) from the circle. This distance can be shortened or lengthened according to participants' abilities.
9. If participant cannot form hollow to flick marble, the "shooter" marble can be positioned on ground and propelled by flicking it with the index finger toward the other marbles.
10. Marbles can be placed in front of a wall to eliminate the need for marble recovery. Several marble games are played in this manner.
11. If participant does not have sufficient eye-hand coordination to shoot a marble, one end of a board or ramp can be leaned against a wall or positioned on a stack of books, allowing player to simply roll marbles down board toward other marbles.
12. An adapted version of marbles is the game of "Bounce Eye." Players must stand over group of marbles, with their shooter marbles straight across at eye level. Players try to knock as many marbles out of circle as possible by dropping marble into circle.

Name of Activity: Pinball

Instructional Objective: Given a pinball game, the participant will operate the plunger and release (play) 3 balls, keeping each ball in play for at least 5 seconds, 80% of the time.
Materials: pinball machine
Verbal Cue: "Dorene, play pinball."

Task Analysis:
1. Extend dominant arm outward toward ball release plunger.
2. Grasp knob with dominant hand using pincer grasp.

3. Pull knob out away from table by bending at elbow.
4. Release ball release plunger by extending fingers.
5. Place dominant hand on the flipper button on one side of pinball machine.
6. Place nondominant hand on the flipper button on the other side of pinball machine.
7. Press flipper button to keep ball in play.
8. Play first ball, keeping it in play for at least 5 seconds.
9. Play second ball, keeping it in play for at least 5 seconds.
10. Play third ball, keeping it in play for at least 5 seconds.

Activity Guidelines/Special Adaptations:
1. Initially, guide participant through motions of game by placing a hand on hers to release ball and operate both flippers.
2. Table model pinball games are commercially available.
3. For easily distracted participants, simple games should be used progressing to more elaborate games when proficiency is acquired.
4. Pinball is excellent game for persons who typically do not show an interest in recreational activities. The game is easily operated and elicits several sounds and flashing lights when manipulated. Participants can even learn to watch points being scored.

Name of Activity: Ping Pong (Table Tennis)

Instructional Objective: Given a ping pong table, paddle, ball, and another player, the participant will serve the ball over the net to her opponent's side of the table, and hit it for a second time after it is returned to her, 50% of the time.

Materials: ping pong table, 2 ping pong paddles, 1 ping pong ball
Verbal Cue: "Lillian, play ping pong."

Task Analysis:
1. Stand at one end of table with feet parallel and shoulder width apart.
2. Extend dominant hand toward ping pong paddle.
3. Grasp handle of paddle with dominant hand using palmar grasp.
4. Extend nondominant hand toward ping pong ball.
5. Grasp ball in nondominant hand using palmar grasp.
6. Raise nondominant hand with ball 6 inches above table top by bending at elbow keeping palm parallel to floor.
7. Raise dominant hand with racket to same height.
8. Flex wrist until paddle is perpendicular to table.
9. Position ball directly in front of paddle.

10. To serve, release grasp on ball by extending fingers allowing ball to bounce on table.
11. Swing paddle forward as ball bounces upward to hit ball across net.
12. Attend to ball as it bounces across table.
13. Wait for ball to be returned by opponent.
14. Position paddle behind oncoming ball.
15. As ball approaches, swing paddle for second time to return ball to opponent's side of table.
16. Continue playing game until participant or opponent misses shot and it is necessary to serve once again.

Activity Guidelines/Special Adaptations:
1. Provide siderails 1½ inches high and 1 inch wide across length of table to avoid ping pong ball rolling off table.
2. Adapted ping pong game can be played requiring ball to travel *through* a net made by piece of string instead of over the net.
3. A ping pong ball dispenser is commercially available that can hold up to 120 ping pong balls. The dispenser releases a ball for 25 cents. Participant can learn money spending concepts; the dispenser can facilitate better care of equipment.
4. A Fenodesis splint can be used as a brace for a paralyzed hand with effective wrist extensors.
5. A bi-handled paddle that allows broader and freer movements has been designed to assist players with upper extremity involvement.
6. Serve changes each time five points are scored between players. A point is scored each time a player fails to return the ball.
7. Players should learn to call, "out" if the ball is hit off the table by the other player.
8. Initially, a larger ball (i.e., Nerf ball or balloon) can be used to slow down the pace of the game. The rules can be changed to allow a ball to bounce more than one time before it has to be returned to opponent.

Name of Activity: Tic-Tac-Toe

Instructional Objective: Given a tic-tac-toe block and a set of "X" and "O" markers, the participant, taking turns with another player, will place her markers in the game board squares until 3 consecutive markers, vertically, horizontally, or diagonally are obtained, 80% of the time.

Materials: tic-tac-toe block, a set "X" and "O" markers (5 in each set)

Verbal Cue: "Ceil, play tic-tac-toe."

Task Analysis:
1. Extend dominant arm downward toward markers.
2. Grasp one marker using pincer grasp.
3. Extend dominant arm toward tic-tac-toe block.
4. Place marker on 1 of the empty squares.
5. Release grasp by extending fingers.
6. Wait for opponent to take turn.
7. Place second marker on empty square.
8. Place third marker on empty square to facilitate blocking opponent's line.
9. Continue alternating with opponent until 3 consecutive squares, vertically, horizontally, or diagnonially, are obtained by one set of markers to obtain tic-tac-toe.

Activity Guidelines/Special Adaptations:
1. Tic-tac-toe board should be large and secured to the table; for motor impaired players, the markers should be made large and thick for easy manipulation.
2. A tic-tac-toe board outlined in heavy yarn can be adapted for visually imparied players. The markers can be made of two different textures such as sandpaper and felt.
3. Tic-tac-toe ring toss games can be made or purchased commercially.
4. Higher level players can play tic-tac-toe on paper, with paint, etc. Participants can also use different colored markers to improve color discrimination skills.
5. Participants should learn to call "tic-tac-toe" immediately following the placement of the third consecutive marker to win game.

MOTOR GAMES

Name of Activity: Arm Wrestle

Instructional Objective: Given an opponent, the participant will pull the opponent's hand from a perpendicular position to a horizontal position on the table top (against the opponent's force pulling participant's hand in opposite direction), 50% of the time.
Materials: another player
Verbal Cue: "Jerry, have an arm wrestle."

Task Analysis:
1. Sit facing opponent at table.
2. Extend dominant arm to midline of body.
3. Bend dominant arm at elbow until arm is perpendicular to table.
4. Place elbow on table in front of body.

5. Extend dominant hand toward opponent's hand (who has positioned arm in same manner.)
6. Place palm of dominant hand against opponent's dominant hand.
7. Grasp opponent's hand using palmar grasp.
8. Place dominant arm against opponent's dominant arm.
9. On "go" apply downward pressure to opponent's hand, pulling it toward nondominant side of body.
10. Continue applying downward pressure against opponent's arm until one player weakens.
11. Pull opponent's hand downward until it is horizontal to table top to win arm wrestle.

Activity Guidelines/Special Adaptations:
1. Make sure that participant and opponent are evenly matched in size and strength to avoid injury.
2. Instruct participants to hold dominant upper arm with nondominant hand to help stabilize the dominant arm.
3. A rubber substance or towel can be placed under participants arms to avoid elbow sliding.
4. It is recommended, whenever possible, to have participants arm wrestle with each arm to build forearm and bicep strength equally on each limb.
5. Isometric contraction (force against force) is an excellent means to build body strength. Arm wrestling utilizes this exercise concept.

Name of Activity: Follow the Leader

Instructional Objective: Given 2 or more players and a group leader, the participant will follow in line doing whatever the leader does, 80% of the time.

Materials: 2 or more players

Verbal Cue: "Paul, follow the leader."

Task Analysis:
1. Stand single file behind and facing back of leader.
2. Attend to each movement that leader makes.
3. Leader flies like an airplane: extend arms outward away from each side of body.
4. Walk behind leader in this manner until leader does another action.

Activity Guidelines/Special Adaptations:
1. Motor impaired participants can do nonlocomotor movements such as whistling, winking, singing, tapping, etc.

2. Initially, demonstrate many different movements that can be used when playing follow the leader (e.g., elephant, jump, walk and clap, etc.)
3. This is a good game to play with group on an outing, in park, or picnic since no equipment is necessary.
4. Add additional supervising assistants to game to prompt motor impaired or lower functioning participants on a one-to-one basis.
5. Begin game with fewer movements leading to more movements as participants become more proficient.
6. If player fails to perform give action, he leaves spot in line and joins end of same line, instead of being out. Allow leader to lead for only a few minutes and then send him to end of line. Next in line becomes new leader. In this manner, all get opportunity to lead.

Name of Activity: Hand Slap

Instructional Objective: Given 2 participants, the participant will slap the top of his opponent's hands before the opponent moves his hands away, 25% of the time.

Materials: 2 players

Verbal Cue: "Bea, play hand slap."

Task Analysis:
1. Stand/sit facing opponent, feet shoulder's width apart.
2. Extend both arms forward to midline of body, fingers extended outward.
3. Rotate hands until palms face upward.
4. Spread hands apart 6 inches.
5. Wait for opponent to lay palms on top of participant's hands (palms on palms).
6. Participant whose palms are underneath—quickly rotate wrists, turning thumbs inward to slap opponent's hands.
7. Simultaneously, participant whose palms are on top attempts to remove hand before being slapped.
8. Continue hand rotation until palms are face downward and on top of opponent's or have touched opponent's hands in slapping motion.

Activity Guidelines/Special Adaptations:
1. This motor game is an excellent way to improve eye-hand coordination.
2. At first game can be played slapping only one hand, then progress to slapping with both hands concurrently.
3. It should be stressed that it is not necessary to hit opponent's hands with great force; a light tap is sufficient to score.

Games   175

Name of Activity: Hopscotch

Instructional Objective: Given a pebble and hopscotch square, the participant will throw pebble into first square, hop into second through eighth squares, pick up pebble, return, throw pebble into second square, hop into square 1 and 3 through 8. Participant will then repeat process until pebble has been thrown into all 8 squares and he has correctly hopped into squares without stepping on any lines, 50% of the time.

Materials: hopscotch block (8 consecutively lined 1-foot squares, with fourth and fifth squares and seventh and eighth squares side by side, 1-inch pebble or button.

Verbal Cue: "Suzie, play hopscotch."

Task Analysis:
1. Extend dominant arm downward toward pebble.
2. Grasp pebble firmly using pincer grasp.
3. Stand facing hopscotch square 1 foot from base of diagram.
4. Extend dominant arm forward directly over first square.
5. Rotate dominant hand until palm is facing downward.
6. Extend fingers of dominant hand to release pebble into block 1.
7. Lower body by bending at knees.
8. Bend at nondominant knee to position foot behind body.
9. Extend arms forward in front of body.
10. Swing arms backward.
11. Hop forward on dominant leg over square 1 into square 2 by extending at knee.
12. Hop into square 3 without stepping on any lines.
13. Jump into squares 4 and 5, by placing one foot in each square.
14. Hop into square 6 without stepping on any lines.
15. Jump into squares 7 and 8, by placing one foot in each square.
16. Turn and continue process in opposite direction.
17. Stop in Square 2, maintaining hopping position
18. Extend dominant arm downward toward pebble in square 1.
19. Grasp pebble using pincer grasp.
20. Hop into square 1.
21. Hop out of hopscotch diagram.
22. Release pebble into square 2.
23. Hop into square 1.
24. Hop over square 2 into block 3.
25. Continue entire process until pebble has been tossed into all 8 squares.

Activity Guidelines/Special Adaptations:
1. Use bean bag or larger stone to toss into hopscotch squares for easier tossing. If a stone is used, it should be flat so it does not roll from box.
2. Outline hopscotch square with string on grass to reduce chance of injury if participant falls.
3. Participant can step into the appropriate squares, instead of hopping, to simplify activity. As participant becomes more proficient, she may begin to hop on one foot into the squares.
4. Letters, words, colors, etc. can be substituted for numbers in the blocks, if preferred.
5. It would appear that enlarging the squares would make it easier to hop without stepping on any lines. Larger squares, however, make hopping from one square to the next a more difficult task for many participants.
6. This is an excellent game to improve eye-hand-foot coordination, agility, and dynamic balance.

Name of Activity: Jump Rope

Instructional Objective: Given a jump rope, the participant will turn the rope and jump through it 2 consecutive times, 80% of the time.
Materials: jump rope
Verbal Cue: "Sybil, jump rope."

Task Analysis:
1. Extend both arms downard toward jump rope handles.
2. Grasp handles using palmar grasp.
3. Hold jump rope handles waist high 8 inches from sides of body.
4. Swing jump rope over head by rotating arms back and in circular motion over head back to sides of body.
5. Bend knees as jump rope approaches ground level in front of body.
6. Jump 2 inches off ground to allow jump rope to pass underneath feet 1 time.
7. Jump rope second consecutive time.

Activity Guidelines/Special Adaptations:
1. At first participant can jump a rope that is twirled by two other players. This eliminates the double task of twirling and jumping simultaneously, so as the participant can concentrate exclusively on jumping the rope.
2. Participants having difficulty jumping rope in the standard fashion can merely swing rope back and forth at sides of body and jump over it.

3. Participants having difficulty jumping rope as described above can practice jumping over a still rope stretched and held between two people.
4. Have a more proficient individual jump with the participant verbally cueing her to "jump, jump."
5. To practice the motor skill of jumping, have participant jump up and down in place.
6. Participants need to be ambulatory to perform this skill.
7. Jumping rope is an excellent activity to improve dynamic balance, eye-hand-foot coordination and to increase arm, leg, and shoulder strength.

Name of Activity: Kickball

Instructional Objective: Given a kickball and a team of 4 or more players positioned in the outfield, the participant will kick the ball in fair territory and run to first base without being tagged or thrown out, 25% of the time.

Materials: large playground ball or volleyball, 4 bases 45 feet apart, 4 or more players

Verbal Cue: "Patti, kick the ball."

Task Analysis:
1. Stand at home plate facing outfield with feet shoulder's width apart.
2. Attend to ball as it approaches home plate.
3. Bend knee of dominant leg to raise foot 6 inches off ground.
4. Continue to bend at knee until foot is positioned behind body.
5. Swing dominant foot forward by extending at knee until toe makes contact with approaching ball.
6. Follow through until instep of foot or toe is perpendicular to ground and makes contact with ball.
7. Kick ball into fair territory.
8. Bend right knee raising foot 6 inches off ground.
9. Extend right knee moving foot forward 1 step toward first base.
10. Place right foot on ground shifting weight to right side of body.
11. Bend left knee raising foot 6 inches off ground.
12. Extend left knee moving left foot forward 1 step toward first base.
13. Continue running until batter reaches first base safely.

Activity Guidelines/Special Adaptations:
1. To simplify activity, make field smaller with bases closer together. Bases can be painted bright red for easy location.
2. Use large, soft ball such as beach ball to make it easier to kick.

3. Have yellers or coaches standing at each base to guide visually impaired participants.
4. Practice rolling, throwing, catching, and kicking balls as separate leadup activities before participants actually play game.
5. Individuals in wheelchairs can kick ball while sitting in chairs and should practice kicking a ball being rolled to them.
6. Kickball is an excellent leadup game to softball, since rules and ideas of each game are similar.

Name of Activity: Parachute Play

Instructional Objective: Given 15 or more players arranged in a 10-foot circle and a parachute spread out on the ground inside the circle, the participant will help to make a mushroom by raising the parachute over her head and then lowering it to waist level, 80% of the time.

Materials: parachute, 15 or more players

Verbal Cue: "Mary, lift the parachute over your head."

Task Analysis:
1. Stand facing inside of circle, feet parallel and shoulder-width apart.
2. Bend knees until body is in squatting position.
3. Extend arms downward toward outer edge of parachute.
4. Grasp parachute using palmar grasp.
5. Extend knees until body is perpendicular to ground.
6. Lift parachute to waist level by bending at elbows.
7. Continue raising arms until parachute is above head height and arms are fully extended.
8. Bend at elbows to lower parachute to waist level to form muschroom.

Activity Guidelines/Special Adaptations:
1. If parachute is too large, heavy, or not available, participants can use a bed sheet to form the mushroom.
2. Size of parachute should be appropriate for number of participants involved.
3. Begin activity with no more than 5 participants in a circle and, with proficiency, involve more players, one at a time.
4. If participant has difficulty grasping edge of parachute, velcro or rope loops can be attached to edge of parachute.
5. Parachute play is an excellent gross motor recreational activity for large groups.
6. Stress the importance of all participants raising and lowering the parachute at the same time to form mushroom. It is recommended that supervising assistants be evenly distributed around the parachute to assist with this activity.

7. Many exercises and games can be implemented using a parachute (e.g., balls placed on top of parachute and flipped into holes using the parachute; participants run underneath it and attempt to get out before parachute lands; circle games; guess the animal formed by players underneath the parachute. Excellent activities for developing upper arm and shoulder strength, eye-hand coordination, and socialization skills.
8. Parachutes can be purchased commercially. Be sure the parachute is made of a strong washable nylon fabric for durability. They are available in 6-foot to 24-foot diameters with brightly striped patterns.
9. Parachute play and dance records are available with instruction manual and instructions on the record.

Name of Activity: Simon Says

Instructional Objective: Given a group of 3 or more players and a leader to act as "Simon," the participant will do what "Simon" commands, but only when the command is preceded with "Simon says," 80% of the time.

Materials: 4 or more players

Verbal Cue: "Steven, Simon says, put your hands on your head."

Task Analysis:
1. Stand facing player designated as "Simon."
2. Attend to command given by "Simon."
3. Observe if command was preceded with "Simon says."
4. If command is preceded with "Simon says," perform appropriate action (i.e., "Simon says, put hands on head")
5. Extend both arms over head.
6. Bend arms at elbows placing hands on top of head.
7. If command is not preceded with "Simon says," stand still and do not obey command.
8. Attend to next command.

Activity Guidelines/Special Adaptations:
1. The role of "Simon" as a group leader can be demonstrated in several games.
2. Gear commands to physical ability level of participants. *Do not ask them* to perform actions they are not capable of doing.
3. Use signs for hearing impaired players.
4. Simon says will reinforce the importance of good listening skills and following directions.
5. Parts of body can be learned during implementation of this activity. As a leadup activity, before playing game, call out a part of the body

(i.e., knee, nose) and have participants place a hand on the designated body part.
6. Simon Says can be a teaching activity for left, right, up, down, forward, backward, etc., as well as body parts.
7. The leader can make the game more confusing by going through the actions each time a command is given, even if the command is not preceded with "Simon says."

Name of Activity: Tag

Instructional Objective: Given 3 or more players, the participants will run away from the person who is "it" to avoid being tagged and will reach the safety base, 50% of the time.
Materials: 3 or more players, base (i.e., tree, floor marker)
Verbal Cue: "Paulene, play tag."

Task Analysis:
1. Locate person who is "it" and safety base.
2. Bend dominant leg at knee raising foot 4 inches from ground.
3. Place foot 1 step forward onto ground by extending leg at knee.
4. Bend nondominant leg at knee raising foot 4 inches from ground.
5. Place foot 1 step forward onto ground by extending leg at knee.
6. Continue to run away from "it" player and toward safety base.
7. Arrive at safety base and stop running.

Activity Guidelines/Special Adaptations:
1. Have participants practice gently tagging others on shoulder or back to make certain participants understand this concept before beginning the tag game.
2. Outline a space with rope to reinforce the concept of "out"; anyone that is tagged is "out" and will remain in that area. Players do not necessarily have to be out, they can also be "it" and try to tag others or can be freed by others from "out" area.
3. Participants can learn to play several different types of tag. There are literally hundreds of variations of the game (i.e., freeze tag, flag tag, nose and toe tag, Japanese tag just to name a few). In freeze tag, a player that is tagged must "freeze" until another player comes to the rescue. "It" player must pull a flag from player's back pocket in flag tag. As long as a player is holding his nose with one hand and a foot with his other, he cannot be tagged in nose and toe tag. The "it" players must hold one hand on the part of the body that was touched when he was tagged in Japanese tag.
4. It is recommended that playing area be clearly marked off in order

for participants to know exactly where they can and cannot run. Boundaries will ensure that players do not wander off alone.

Name of Activity: Tetherball

Instructional Objective: Given a tetherball, pole, and 2 players, the participant will stand within the designated boundaries and hit the ball, winding the rope and ball in the opposite direction of his opponent, at least twice around the pole, 80% of the time.

Materials: tetherball, pole (10 feet above ground), 2 players

Verbal Cue: "Jeffrey, play tetherball."

Task Analysis:
1. Stand in designated boundaries of tetherball court, feet shoulder-width apart.
2. As tetherball approaches, extend fingers of dominant hand to expose palm in slapping position.
3. Position arm at side of body, hand at shoulder height, elbow bent.
4. Swing arm foward at shoulder until open hand makes contact with ball.
5. Continue hit with follow through.
6. Reposition arm to hitting position.
7. As ball approaches for second time, swing arm forward to hit ball second time around pole.
8. Continue hitting ball until rope and ball have wound completely around pole.

Activity Guidelines/Special Adaptations:
1. Playing time can be shortened by shortening the rope so that the ball will not have to be wrapped around the pole as many times.
2. Use baseball glove, tennis racket, or heavy paddle to hit ball instead of using hand to simplify activity.
3. Person in wheelchair can participate if pole is lowered and rope shortened.
4. Tetherball is an excellent game to improve visual tracking skills and eye-hand coordination.
5. As a leadup activity, a tetherball of volleyball can be suspended from the ceiling with cord. Participants can practice hitting the ball continuously by themselves.
6. Player's hand does not necessarily have to be open; a clenched fist can be used if desired. Ball will usually move faster around pole if hit with fist and, consequently, players may have to move more quickly to avoid being hit in the head by the approaching ball.

Name of Activity: Tug of War

Instructional Objective: Given a 20-foot piece of rope evenly distributed over a marked center line and an opponent of similar abilities, the participant will grasp one end of the rope and pull the opponent holding the opposite end over the center line, 50% of the time.

Materials: 20-foot piece of rope, marker for center line (i.e., mat, chalk), even number of players on either side

Verbal Cue; "Anne, pull the rope."

Task Analysis:
1. Stand by rope on appropriate side of center line, feet parallel and shoulder-width apart.
2. Extend nondominant arm downward toward rope.
3. Grasp rope firmly using palmar grasp.
4. Extend dominant arm downward toward rope.
5. Hold rope firmly, approximately 2 inches in front of nondominant grasp, using palmar grasp.
6. Lift rope to height just above waist level.
7. Wait for signal to begin tug of war.
8. Pull rope back toward body by bending arms at elbows.
9. Shift weight to dominant leg.
10. Bend nondominant leg at knee, raising foot 4 inches off ground.
11. Place nondominant foot one step backward behind dominant foot to move opponent forward.
12. Shift weight to nondominant leg.
13. Bend dominant leg at knee, raising foot 4 inches from ground.
14. Place dominant foot one step backward behind nondominant foot to move opponent 2 feet forward.
15. Pull rope and step backward to move opponent 3 feet forward.
16. Pull rope and step backward to move opponent 5 feet forward.
17. Pull rope and step backward to move opponent 10 feet forward to win tug of war.

Activity Guidelines/Special Adaptations:
1. In initial stages of participation in tug of war game, use one-on-one competition in order to evenly match strength of participants. With proficiency, place individuals into a team tug of war, encouraging teamwork.
2. During a team tug of war, smaller and weaker participants should stand near the middle of the rope. That team loses whose first player touches or crosses the center line with her foot.
3. Tug of war is an excellent means to develop upper body strength as

well as gross motor coordination, dynamic balance, cooperation, and teamwork.
4. A four-way tug of war rope is available that will include up to forty participants at one time.
5. The diameter of the rope used should be in proportion to the size of the participants' hands.
6. Gloves can be worn to aid grasping of the rope and to prevent hand and finger burns and blisters. Also, several towels can be tied together to replace the rope and reduce injury.
7. The winner or winning team of a tug of war contest is determined when either one team has been pulled across the center line or, when the predetermined time period (i.e., 2 minutes) has elapsed. At that time the team that has pulled the other further across the line is the winning team.
8. "People tug of war" can be played if a rope is unavailable. Each player on a side wraps her arms around the waist of the person in front of her. The front players on each side hold onto each other's arms. All players try to pull the other team across the center line.
9. Because players occasionally fall backwards when the other team gives way to the tug of war rope, the contest must take place in a barrier-free area. Trees, rocks, lamp posts, etc. can be dangerous if located behind players.

Name of Activity: Twister

Instructional Objective: Given a Twister mat spread flat on the floor, game spinner, and another individual to spin the dial, the participant will place a limb on the corresponding space, following instructions of spinner, for 4 consecutive spins, 80% of the time.
Materials: Twister mat, game spinner, 3 or more players
Verbal Cue: "Chet, place your right foot on blue."

Task Analysis:
1. Stand on one side of game mat, with each leg in a different space closest to the end of mat.
2. Wait for individual to spin game dial.
3. Attend to instructions (i.e., place right foot on blue mark).
4. Raise right foot 4 inches off game mat by bending at knee.
5. Position right foot directly above nearest blue mark.
6. Place foot down on center of blue mark by extending at knee to complete first movement.
7. Wait for individual to spin game dial for second time.
8. Attend to instructions.

9. Move limb to appropriate space to complete second consecutive movement.
10. Complete third consecutive movement.
11. Complete fourth consecutive movement.

Activity Guidelines/Special Adaptations:
1. Tie colored markers around participant's right arm and leg to help distinguish between right and left limbs.
2. Game spinner can be omitted by having leader ask participant to complete specific instructions. In this way, leader can watch body position of participant and consciously make the movement easier to enhance success.
3. Teaching rugs that use the same basic ideas as Twister, are available to teach many gross and perceptual motor skills using hands, heels, toes and also, crossing midline activities. Flexibility, dynamic and static balance could be enhanced through participation.
4. Spaces on the Twister mat can be used to teach many concepts, such as letter, number, name, shape, and color discrimination.
5. The game is available commercially or can be homemade. Four persons can play simultaneously. For lower functioning participants, make a game mat consisting of larger and fewer colored spaces.
6. If game is homemade, be sure to use heavy duty vinyl that can easily be cleaned with sponge and water and can fold up for easy storage.

MUSICAL/RHYTHMICAL GAMES

Name of Activity: Farmer in the Dell

Instructional Objective: Given the song "Farmer in the Dell," a group of players arranged in a circle holding hands, and 1 player, "farmer," in the center, the participant will sing and walk around in a circle, walk to the inside of circle when picked as a (wife, child, etc.) by the "farmer," then select "child," 80% of the time.

Materials: 7 or more players

Verbal Cue: "Jenna, sing and play "Farmer in the Dell.""

Task Analysis:
1. Hold other players' hands to each side of body, using palmar grasps, forming circle around "farmer."
2. Turn body 90° to right while holding hands.
3. Sing song and walk around in a circle with other players.
4. Sing "Farmer takes a wife" as "farmer" chooses partner for "wife."
5. Release hand grasps with other players by extending fingers, lowering hands to sides.

6. Walk into center of circle to join "farmer."
7. Continue to sing song as others circle around.
8. Extend dominant arm outward, pointing to another player around circle, taking "child."
9. Continue singing song and playing game until 7 players are selected and standing inside circle.

Activity Guidelines/Special Adaptations:
1. Begin activity with participants arranged in circular formation, holding hands, with one player in center of circle acting as "farmer."
2. Players in center of circle can either point, tap, or call name to select person.
3. Flashcards can be given to newly selected participants, depending on the role they are chosen for (i.e., cat gets cat flashcard).
4. Teacher/leader can be "farmer" standing in center of circle to begin game.
5. Each player selected for role in center, in turn, chooses another player to represent the next character: the farmer in the dell, the farmer in the dell, heigh-o, the derry-o, the farmer in the dell. The farmer takes a wife; the wife takes a child; the child takes a nurse; the nurse takes a dog; the dog takes a cat; the cat takes a rat; the rat takes the cheese; and the cheese stands alone.
6. As the last verse is sung by all players, they can begin to clap their hands and gather around the "cheese." If a new round is started, the "cheese" becomes the new "farmer."

Name of Activity: Home Rhythm Band

Instructional Objective: Given a drum and drumstick, cymbals, steel triangle and rod, bell with handle, rattle, xylophone and mallet, the participant will hit one of the percussion instruments to a simple beat, along with 5 other players, 5 consecutive times, 80% of the time.

Materials: drum and drumstick, cymbals, steel triangle and rod, bell with handle, rattle, and xylophone and mallet

Verbal Cue: "Andy, play the (drum, cymbals, triangle, bell, rattle, xylophone)."

Task Analysis:
To play drum:
1. Extend dominant arm downward toward drumstick, palm faced down.
2. Grasp drumstick firmly using palmar grasp.
3. Bend at elbow, raising drumstick to chest level.
4. Position drumstick directly above drum head.

5. Extend at elbow, lowering drumstick to drum head, striking drum 1 time to first beat.
6. Hit drum second time to second beat.
7. Hit drum third time to third beat.
8. Hit drum fourth time to fourth beat.
9. Hit drum fifth time to fifth consecutive beat.

Activity Guidelines/Special Adaptations:
1. Drumstick, steel rod, bell handle, mallet, etc. can be enlarged by wrapping with foam rubber and/or tape for easier manipulation.
2. If participant must strike the percussion instrument with a mallet, etc., make sure instrument is positioned at a comfortable distance away from musician, eliminating an uncomfotable reach or cramped strike.
3. Initially, participants should be concerned with keeping time to simple beat; with proficiency, musicians can practice making different sounds by striking different keys or locations on instrument.
4. Any jar or squeeze bottle filled with sand, dried peas, marbles, etc. can be used to produce other sounds in home rhythm band.
5. Participant does not necessarily have to use arms and hands to participate in percussion instrument band. Head, foot, ankle, elbow etc. can be used to strike instrument. Also, a felt or leather bracelet with bells sewn on it can be worn on wrist or ankle. This is an excellent way to combine music and movement.
6. Participation in a percussion instrument band will improve eye-hand coordination, muscular strength, attending skills, and facilitate social skill development.
7. Most people love to play and listen to music. Participants should be encouraged to make their own music to express themselves physically, release pent-up energies, and to be creative.

Name of Activity: Hot Potato

Instructional Objective: Given a group of players arranged in a circle, a beanbag, and music, the participant will receive the beanbag from another player and pass it on to the next player before the music stops, 80% of the time.

Materials: 3 or more players, record player (tape deck, piano), record (tape), beanbag

Verbal Cue: "Charlotte, pass the hot potato."

Task Analysis:
1. Sit in circle.
2. Music begins.
3. Attend to music and player with beanbag.

4. Attend to beanbag being passed around circle.
5. When player on right receives beanbag, rotate 90° at hips to face other player.
6. Extend arms forward toward beanbag.
7. Grasp beanbag using palmar grasps.
8. Quickly rotate 180° at hips to face player on left.
9. Extend arms forward toward player's extended arms.
10. Release beanbag into player's hands, before music stops, by extending fingers.

Activity Guidelines/Special Adaptations:
1. A ball, sock, or any other easily grasped object can be used instead of beanbag.
2. This activity can be played in either a seated or standing position.
3. Motor impaired participants unable to receive and pass "hot potato" can merely tap object as another player carries it to them.
4. Game can be played by removing those who are left holding "hot potato" when music stops, or by allowing them to remain in game. Players caught holding potato can assist with starting and stopping of music.
5. Before game begins, it should be emphasized that potato is "hot," therefore, must be passed on quickly.

Name of Activity: Limbo

Instructional Objective: Given 2 players, each holding an end of a 5-foot long stick at participant's chest level, the participant will walk under the stick by bending backward at waist without touching the stick, 80% of the time.

Materials: 5-foot long stick, 3 or more players
Verbal Cue: "Gregory, walk under the stick."

Task Analysis:
1. Stand directly in front center of stick facing it, feet shoulder-width apart.
2. Attend to stick raised to chest level.
3. Bend at knees lowering body toward ground.
4. Bend backward at waist lowering upper body.
5. Bend neck backward to lower head.
6. Extend at dominant knee to slide foot forward.
7. Slide nondominant foot forward until parallel with dominant foot.
8. Slide on feet taking second step forward until body positioned below stick.

9. Continue sliding in this manner until entire body has passed under stick without touching it.
10. Extend at waist to stand erect.

Activity Guidelines/Special Adaptations:
1. Activity leader can stand behind participant when walking under stick in case participant loses balance and falls backward (players bend backward at waist).
2. Limbo is an excellent large group activity, especially during social gatherings. Many will enjoy anxiously waiting in line until it is their turn. Music can accompany activity.
3. Game can continue by lowering limbo stick after each successful attempt. As game progresses, activity will get more difficult.
4. Player who does not safely walk under stick without touching it can get back in line to wait for next attempt, or can become new limbo stick holder.
5. Participant must continue to bend at waist if upper body is not low enough to safely walk under stick.
6. If participant is unable to bend backward at waist to lower upper body, bending forward at waist should be permissable.
7. Individuals in wheelchairs can also participate. Have them attempt to travel underneath stick at neck height, then chest height. These individuals must bend at neck, then at waist to safely pass under stick.

Name of Activity: London Bridge

Instructional Objective: Given the song "London Bridge," the participant will sing and make a hand bridge with another player and catch 3 other players by making bridge fall, 80% of the time.

Materials: 5 or more players

Verbal Cue: "Betsy, make a bridge and sing along."

Task Analysis:
To build bridge:
1. Stand facing other player.
2. Keeping arms extended, raise arms upward and outward until palms meet with other player's hands.
3. Interlock hands with other player by curling fingers through spaces of other player's fingers until participant's fingers touch back of other player's hand.
4. Maintain above stance allowing players to pass under bridge until bridge falls down catching one player.

To catch player:
5. Keeping hands clasped with other player, lower arms concurrently as one player is passing directly under bridge, until arms are surrounding caught player at waist.
6. Rock caught player by swaying arms first to one side and then to the other side of caught player's body.
7. Release hand grips by extending fingers and lowering arms toward body making bridge fall to catch first player.
8. Raise bridge.
9. Catch second player by making bridge fall.
10. Catch third player.
11. Caught players become part of bridge until all players have been caught.

Activity Guidelines/Special Adaptations:
1. This musical game is an excellent facilitator of social skill development, as all players must work cooperatively to form bridge. After player is caught, she must stand behind player forming bridge, wrapping her arms around that player's waist.
2. To make game more realistic for participants, name of bridge can be changed from London Bridge to another name of bridge in players' hometown (e.g., in New York: Brooklyn Bridge).
3. Players unfamiliar with game can be paired with more competent individuals to form bridge.
4. Players should be encouraged to sing along after they have learned motions of game. Participants physically unable to play can be singers, so that all may participate in one way or another.
5. Players forming bridge should be encouraged to be gentle when catching player, making sure not to hit player's head as bridge falls.
6. Several verses can be sung: London Bridge is falling down, . . . , . . . , . . . , . . . , My fair lady; Build it up with iron bars, etc.

Name of Activity: Musical Chairs

Instructional Objective: Given a group of players, and chairs numbering one less than participants arranged in a circle with backs of chairs toward inside of circle, and music that can be turned on and off, the participant will walk around the chairs to the music, sit down in chair when the music stops, 80% of the time.

Materials: record player, record, (or piano), 5 or more players, chairs numbering one less than number of players

Verbal Cue: "Sarah, find a seat when the music stops."

Task Analysis:
1. Listen for music to begin.
2. Walk around chairs in clockwise direction as music plays.
3. Sit in closest chair as soon as music stops.
4. Participant who is unable to find vacant chair must leave circle.
5. Remove chiar from circle.
6. Continue to play until one participant (winner) is remaining.

Activity Gudielines/Special Adaptations:
1. Game may be played by nonambulatory participants by merely outlining areas on floor with tape that participants move to when music stops.
2. A cassette tape player can be used that allows a participant to stop and start the music by merely pressing button on the deck.
3. Players who have left the game should be encouraged to cheer or otherwise maintain interest in the game. A player who is out can control the music or can remain seated without remvoing a chair so as not to be eliminated.
4. Players should be encouraged to march with their knees raised high to avoid running around the chairs.
5. No two players may occupy same chair at same time. If this occurs, participant on bottom (first one seated) remains.

CARD GAMES

Name of Activity: Concentration

Instructional Objective: Given a standard size deck of playing cards, each card face down on the table, the participant will draw any two cards from the spread out pack, attempting to draw 2 cards that match, 80% of the time.
Materials: standard size deck of playing cards, 1 or more players
Verbal Cue: "Christopher, pick two cards that match."

Task Analysis:
1. Extend dominant hand downward toward cards face down on table.
2. Position hand directly above desired card to be drawn.
3. Grasp card using pincer grasp.
4. Rotate wrist turning card over, exposing face of card.
5. Place card face up on table top by extending fingers.
6. Draw second card.
7. Determine whether or not 2 cards match.
8. Turn cards face down to original position if cards do not match.

9. If cards match, pick up both cards using pincer grasp.
10. Release cards onto table in front of self.

Activity Guidelines/Special Adaptations:
1. Initially, matching cards can be arranged adjacent to each other to facilitate success in matching cards.
2. Game can be played with fewer cards face down on table to simplify activity.
3. Use any "pair" card game such as Old Maid to improve matching skills.
4. Use picture or color "pairs" cards to improve matching skills within context of a game.
5. When a matched pair is made, participant will take another turn until the cards he draws do not form a pair. Each player always draws 2 cards, 1 at a time.
6. Remember, the object of the game is to win the greatest number of cards by drawing pairs (e.g., 2 aces, 2 three's, 2 jacks, etc.).
7. Stress the importance of attending to other player's draws—watch where Christopher puts the king and five. An excellent game to improve memory, this is why the game is called "Concentration."
8. Jokers can be used as wild cards. Any other card selected will form a match with a joker.
9. This card game can facilitate social skills development since any number of players can play at one time.

Name of Activity: I Doubt It

Instructional Objective: Given a standard size deck of playing cards, all evenly dealt to players, the participant will lay the appropriate card(s) face down or another bluff card(s) if she does not have that card rank, when it is her turn, 80% of the time.
Materials: standard size deck of playing cards, 3 or more players
Verbal Cue: "Fanny, lay down your two's (three's, four's, etc.)."

Task Analysis:
1. Hold cards in nondominant hand.
2. Identify card ranks.
3. Arrange cards in hand by matching same rank cards in sequential order.
4. Attend to cards to see if two's are in hand.
5. Play all two's in hand onto table face down.
6. Say "(*number*) two's."

7. If no two's in hand, play another card(s) face down and say "*(number)* two's" to bluff other players.
8. Wait to hear if another player doubts call.
9. If no player doubts call, next player to left plays three's or bluff card(s).
10. If player doubts call and if cards played were two's, player that doubted call picks up all cards from center of table.
11. If player doubts call and if cards player were not two's but were bluff cards, participant that played bluff card(s) picks up all cards from center of table.
12. Continue game by playing cards in rank order, in turn, until 1 player gets rid of all cards.

Activity Guidelines/Special Adaptations:
1. For participants having difficulty holding cards in hand, playing card holders are available that hold standard card hands and expose all card faces to player. Cost is less than $3.
2. This card game can facilitate social skills development since any number of players, up to 13, can play at one time.
3. Remember, the object of the game is to be the first to get rid of all one's cards.
4. The first player to put down cards must discard two's, next player three's, next four's, up to kings and aces and then back to two's.
5. Each player must play at least 1 card when it is her turn whether or not she has a card of the appropriate rank.

Name of Activity: Old Maid

Instructional Objective: Given a deck of "Old Maid" cards, the participant will draw 1 card from the player to her left and lay her paired cards on the table when it is her turn, 80% of the time.

Materials: deck of "Old Maid" cards or standard size deck of playing cards (queen of clubs omitted), 2 or more players

Verbal Cue: "Donna, pick up a card and lay down your pairs."

Task Analysis:
1. Hold cards in nondominant hand.
2. Arrange cards in hand by paris.
3. Remove all pairs from hand and place them on table concurrently with other players.
4. Draw card from the hand of player to left.
5. Look for pair.
6. If pair is formed, lay pair down on table.

7. If no pair is formed, add card to those in hand.
8. Hold cards in hand for player on right to draw card.
9. Continue playing game by drawing 1 card at a time and forming pairs, until all pairs have been laid down except queen.
10. Player holding queen is Old Maid.

Activity Guidelines/Special Adaptations:
1. As a leadup activity, have participants practice forming pairs in their hands and discarding them onto the table.
2. Use any "pairs" card game, such as "Concentration," to improve matching skills.
3. At first, use picture or color "pairs" cards to improve matching skills within context of a game.
4. Remember, the object of the game is to form and discard pairs, not to be left with the queen card at game's end.
5. This card game can facilitate social skill development since any number of players can play at one time.

Name of Activity: Slap Jack

Instructional Objective: Given a standard size deck of playing cards, all evenly dealt to players, the participant will slap the jack after it is played by another player or himself, 50% of the time.

Materials: standard size deck of playing cards, 3 to 8 players

Verbal Cue: "Nolan, slap the jack."

Task Analysis:
1. Extend dominant arm downward toward stack of cards on table.
2. Grasp top card using pincer grasp.
3. Play card onto table, face up.
4. Continue playing cards until jack appears face up.
5. Extend dominant hand toward played jack.
6. Lower hand palm faced downward onto top of jack before other players.
7. Pick up stack of cards by bending at elbow.
8. Place stack of cards onto table in front of self.
9. Continue playing cards and slapping jacks as they are played to center of table until one player has won all cards.

Activity Guidelines/Special Adaptations:
1. If participant is unable to slap the jack as it is played to the center, door bell buzzers can be used, requiring a simple finger movement after jack is played.

2. A similar game can be played utilizing all picture cards as slap cards which makes game more interesting. In this manner, game will be more lively and involve less waiting.
3. Game can be altered to make any card a slap card to facilitate identification of several different cards.
4. Participants should be paired as equally as possible in the areas of conceptual, gross motor, eye-hand coordination, and reflex skills.
5. Larger playing cards can be used for easier manipulation and for visually impaired participants. Larger cards will also give players larger surface to slap.
6. Remember, the object of the game is to slap jacks as they are played to center of table before other players do, to win all the cards.

Name of Activity: War

Instructional Objective; Given a standard size deck of playing cards, all dealt out evenly and stacked face down in front of players, the participant will play one card at a time simultaneously with another player, identify the higher ranked card and play until one player has won all the cards, 80% of the time.

Materials: standard size deck of playing cards, 2 or more players

Verbal Cue: "Dick, play your top card."

Task Analysis:
1. Extend dominant hand downward toward pile of cards.
2. Grasp top card using pincer grasp.
3. Play card face up on table simultaneously with another player.
4. Determine higher ranked card.
5. If card is of higher rank, extend dominant hand toward 2 cards in center of table.
6. Pick up cards from center of table using pincer grasp.
7. Remove cards from center of table to participant's playing area.
8. Release cards onto table in front of self by extending fingers.
9. If other player's card is of higher rank, wait for player to remove cards.
10. Continue playing cards, one at a time until one player has all cards.

Activity Guidelines/Special Adaptations:
1. War can be used to improve rank order identification skills.
2. When both cards played are of same rank, "War" is declared. Originally played cards are left on table and each play draws additional card, face down. Then another card is played face up, and the higher ranking card of last 2 played wins all 6 cards.

3. Larger playing cards can be used for easier manipulation and for visually impaired participants.
4. Remember, object of game is to win all cards. Aces are considered highest ranked cards.
5. War is excellent activity for 2 players, but more can play at a time. This card game is highly recommended for persons lacking good card skills. War only requires players to determine higher ranked card of 2, making it one of the simplest card games to play.

Chapter 9
OBJECT MANIPULATION

Toys and other objects are effective tools that can be utilized to encourage play and improve manipulatory/eye-hand coordination skills in children as well as adults. Manipulatory objects are appropriate for children as the simplest form of leisure participation (e.g., Busy Box, jack-in-the-box); and some are appropriate for adolescents and adults (e.g., frisbee, vending machine). Since there is a large variety of objects commercially available, there are several criteria for selection that should be recognized including: specific purpose and function of object, versatility, safety, cost, and potential to stimulate the individual, just to name a few. The manipulation of objects should be a part of every individual's leisure repertoire, as it can help the person master specific skills and allow for creativity. Additionally, object manipulation can act as a leadup to participation in various hobbies, sports, and games, since most of these require the manipulation of objects.

The object manipulation skills in this chapter include:

Age Level*	Objects	Page
	BLOCKS	
C	Build Block Tower	198
C	Load Blocks into Toy Truck	199
	BUCKET AND SHOVEL	
C	Fill Bucket Using Shovel	200
C	Build Sand Castle	201
	BUSY BOX	
C	Push Beeper	202
C	Slide Door	203
C	Turn Dial	204
	CRAYONS	
C	Color Picture	205
	FRISBEE	
C/A	Throw Frisbee	205
C/A	Catch Frisbee	206
	HANDGRIPPER	
C/A	Squeeze Handgripper	207
	HULA-HOOP	
C	Spin Hula-Hoop On Floor	207
C	Swing Hula-Hoop On Arm	208
C	Twirl Hula-Hoop Around Waist	209

* C, Indicates chronologically age-appropriate for child; A, Indicates chronologically age-appropriate for adolescent and adult; C/A, Indicates chronologically age-appropriate for child, adolescent, and adult.

	JACK-IN-THE-BOX	
C	Stuff Jack-In-The-Box	210
	Wind Jack-In-The Box	211
	MARBLES	
C	Roll Marble	212
C	Shoot Marble	213
	MR. BUBBLE	
C	Open Bottle	214
C	Blow Bubble	215
	MULTIPURPOSE BALL	
C	Roll Ball	215
C	Kick Ball	216
C	Throw Ball	217
	SCISSORS	
C/A	Open/Close Scissors (Cutting Movement)	218
C/A	Cut Paper On Straight Line	219
C/A	Cut Out Picture	219
	SLINKY	
C	Stretch Slinky	220
C	Walk Slinky Down Steps	220
	TELEPHONE	
C/A	Answer Telephone	222
A	Deposit Money in Pay Telephone	223
C/A	Dial Phone Number	224
C/A	Talk On Telephone	226
	VENDING MACHINE	
C/A	Use of Vending Machine	227

BLOCKS

Name of Activity: Build Block Tower

Instructional Objective: Given a set of 7 blocks, the participant will stack 2 rows of blocks vertically to build a tower, 80% of the time.
Materials: 7 blocks (6 square, 1 rectangular)
Verbal Cue: "Gilda, build a block tower."

Task Analysis:
1. Extend dominant arm downward toward blocks, palm faced down.
2. Lower dominant arm until palm makes contact with first block.
3. Curl fingers around block.
4. Wrap thumb around block.
5. Apply inward pressure between thumb and fingers to grasp block firmly.
6. Extend elbow, moving dominant arm outward 6 inches away from the other 2 blocks.
7. Extend fingers and thumb of dominant hand, releasing block onto ground.

8. Pick up second block.
9. Position second block directly above first block.
10. Extend fingers and thumb, releasing second block onto top of first block.
11. Pick up third block.
12. Place third block on top of second block.
13. Stack another set of 3 blocks vertically, adjacent to first stack.
14. Extend dominant arm downward toward rectangular block, palm faced down.
15. Lower dominant arm until palm makes contact with rectangular block.
16. Curl fingers around block.
17. Wrap thumb around block.
18. Apply inward pressure between thumb and fingers to grasp block firmly.
19. Bend elbow, raising block off ground.
20. Position block directly above 2 vertical stacks of blocks.
21. Lower arm until rectangular block makes contact with both stacks.
22. Extend fingers and thumb, releasing rectangular block onto top of both stacks, forming a tower of blocks.

Activity Guidelines/Special Adaptations:
1. Initially, this activity may be done in a corner using the two sides of the wall for support.
2. Velcro can be attached to the blocks to help hold them together. Magnets can also be used.
3. With proficiency, participant can use more elaborately shaped blocks to build variety of structures. The game of "Blockhead" can be used in conjunction with stacking blocks vertically.
4. At first, blocks with stable stacking shapes, such as squares and rectangles, should be used. Less stable shapes can be gradually introduced.
5. Larger blocks should be placed toward bottom of tower, using progressively smaller blocks near top.
6. Participant can manipulate set of different sized stacking rings and pole as leadup activity to building block tower.

Name of Activity: Load Blocks into Toy Truck

Instructional Objective: Given 3 blocks, the participant will place the blocks into an open-bed toy truck, 80% of the time.
Materials: 3 blocks, open-bed toy truck
Verbal Cue: "Gilda, put the blocks into the truck."

Task Analysis:
1. Position body facing toy truck, arm's reach away.
2. Extend dominant arm downward toward first block, palm faced down.
3. Lower dominant arm until palm makes contact with block.
4. Curl fingers around block.
5. Wrap thumb around block.
6. Apply inward pressure between thumb and fingers to grasp block firmly.
7. Bend elbow, raising block off ground.
8. Position hand holding block directly above open bed of toy truck.
9. Extend fingers and thumb of dominant hand, releasing first block into truck.
10. Pick up second block.
11. Place second block into truck.
12. Pick up third block.
13. Place third block into truck.

Activity Guidelines/Special Adaptations:
1. Size of truck's bed should be large enough so that blocks can easily be placed onto it. Bed should have sides so that blocks do not readily fall out.
2. Appropriate combinational use of two separate toys, as in this activity, has proved to be a significant variable in the play of normal and mentally retarded persons. Participants should be encouraged to use toys in appropriate combinations.
3. This activity can be used in conjunction with replacing blocks in a shoe box or other container or placing them on a shelf.

BUCKET AND SHOVEL

Name of Activity: Fill Bucket Using Shovel

Instructional Objective: Given a bucket, shovel, and sand, the participant will fill the bucket with 2 shovelfuls of sand, 80% of the time.
Materials: bucket, shovel, sand
Verbal Cue: "Leslie, fill the bucket with sand."

Task Analysis:
1. Bend knees, lowering body to ground, kneeling beside sand.
2. Extend dominant arm downward toward shovel, palm faced down.
3. Lower dominant arm until palm makes contact with handle of shovel, shovel faced upward.
4. Curl fingers around handle.

5. Wrap thumb around handle.
6. Apply inward pressure between thumb and fingers to grasp handle firmly.
7. Bend elbow, raising shovel 3 inches off ground.
8. Rotate wrist downward so that shovel forms 45° angle with sand.
9. Extend elbow, lowering scoop of shovel into sand.
10. Rotate wrist upward so that shovel is parallel with ground.
11. Bend elbow, raising shovel 6 inches off ground.
12. Position dominant hand holding shovel directly above center of bucket.
13. Rotate wrist of dominant hand downward 45°, causing sand to fall off shovel into bucket.
14. Dig second shovelful.
15. Dump second shovelful of sand into bucket.

Activity Guidelines/Special Adaptations:
1. This skill can be adapted to digging for worms, planting, or for use in sandbox or on the beach.
2. A scoop made from a plastic one-gallon milk container can be substituted for a shovel. A second container with its top cut off can serve as a bucket.
3. Sand should be dry to make it lighter and easier for participant to dig and carry.
4. Mark should be made on inside of bucket with wide tape or marker, indicating desired level.
5. Filling bucket with glasses of water may be used as a leadup activity to filling bucket with sand.
6. Bucket may be placed on its side with participant pushing sand into it if he has considerable difficulty using a scoop or shovel.

Name of Activity: Build Sand Castle

Instructional Objective: Given a bucket and sand (moistened), the participant will build a sand castle, 80% of the time.

Materials: bucket, sand (moistened)

Verbal Cue: "Leslie, build a sand castle."

Task Analysis:
1. Bend knees, lowering body to ground, kneeling in sand.
2. Scoop sand into bucket (or fill bucket with sand using shovel).
3. Extend nondominant arm outward toward bucket, palm faced down.
4. Lower nondominant arm until palm makes contact with rim of bucket.
5. Curl fingers around rim.

6. Wrap thumb around inner side of rim of bucket.
7. Apply inward pressure between thumb and fingers to grasp rim of bucket firmly.
8. Extend dominant arm downward toward base of bucket, palm faced up.
9. Move dominant arm inward at shoulder, sliding fingers under bottom of bucket, thumb resting on side.
10. Bend both elbows, raising bucket 1 foot off ground.
11. Lower nondominant arm, simultaneously raising dominant arm, causing bucket to tilt so that open end of bucket is facing downward to ground.
12. Lower both arms until rim of bucket makes contact with sand.
13. Move nondominant arm outward at shoulder, sliding hand away from rim of bucket.
14. Extend elbow of dominant arm, applying downward pressure onto bottom of bucket with hand, driving bucket downward into sand.
15. Bend elbow, lifting dominant hand off bottom of bucket.
16. Curl thumb and fingers inward toward palm, forming a fist.
17. Quickly extend elbow of dominant arm, lowering fist onto bottom of bucket, applying downward pressure with fist onto bottom of bucket.
18. Bend elbow, lifting hand off bottom of bucket.
19. Extend both arms downward toward base of bucket, palms faced in.
20. Position hands on either side of base of bucket.
21. Move both arms inward at shoulder until palms make contact with sides of bucket at base.
22. Applying inward pressure between both hands, raise arms straight up at shoulder, lifting bucket up off ground, revealing sand castle formed by bucket.

Activity Guidelines/Special Adaptations:
1. The teacher may moisten the sand with water before the participant fills the bucket with sand.
2. Participant may build a moat around the castle and fill it with water.
3. Participant can use any number of plastic molds that are available to build different shapes for her sand castle.

BUSY BOX

Name of Activity: Push Beeper

Instructional Objective: Given a Busy Box, the participant will push in the beeper, eliciting a sound, 80% of the time.

Materials: Busy Box, beeper
Verbal Cue: "Glenda, push the Busy Box beeper."

Task Analysis:
1. Extend dominant arm downward toward beeper, palm faced down.
2. Lower dominant arm until palm makes contact with beeper.
3. Extend elbow, apply downward pressure onto beeper with hand, eliciting a beep.
4. Bend elbow, raising hand up off beeper.

Activity Guidelines/Special Adaptations:
1. Beeper should be loud enough for participant to hear easily.
2. Teacher may have to explain to participant relationship between pushing the beeper and the resulting sound.
3. If homemade busy box is used, doorbell buzzer and pleasant sounding chimes may be used instead of a beeper. A small Christmas light can be wired to turn on when beeper is pressed.
4. For the cerebral palsied child, an extra large busy box can be made, designed to meet individual needs.
5. Beeper should be of a color that contrasts with background area of Busy Box.

Name of Activity: Slide Door

Instructional Objective: Given a Busy Box, the participant will slide the door open and closed 1 time, 80% of the time.
Materials: Busy Box, sliding door
Verbal Cue: "Glenda, open and close the Busy Box door."

Task Analysis:
1. Extend dominant arm downward toward sliding door, palm faced down, thumb and index finger extended.
2. Lower dominant arm until thumb makes contact with side of door latch.
3. Place index finger onto opposite side of door latch.
4. Apply inward pressure between thumb and index finger to grasp door latch firmly.
5. Move arm at shoulder toward dominant side of body, sliding door open.
6. Move arm at shoulder toward nondominant side of body, sliding door closed.

Activity Guidelines/Special Adaptations:
1. Door should be properly lubricated with paraffin if it does not slide easily.
2. Small velcro or magnetic strips can be used to help participant grasp

door handle. A strip of sandpaper or textured adhesive tape can be applied to handle to provide a better gripping surface.
3. Bright colors or participant's favorite pictures may be taped behind door to encourage participant to open door.

Name of Activity: Turn Dial

Instructional Objective: Given a Busy Box, the participant will turn the dial 3 notches, 80% of the time.
Materials: Busy Box, dial
Verbal Cue: "Glenda, turn the Busy Box dial."

Task Analysis:
1. Extend dominant arm downward toward dial, palm faced down, index finger extended.
2. Lower dominant arm until index finger makes contact with dial.
3. Extend elbow, placing index finger into hole of dial.
4. Lower arm, applying downward pressure onto dial with index finger, turning dial 1 notch in either direction.
5. Continue applying downward pressure onto dial with index finger, turning dial to second notch.
6. Turn dial to third notch.

Activity Guidelines/Special Adaptations:
1. The dial will turn in a clockwise or counterclockwise direction; therefore, downward pressure applied by participant will turn the dial in either direction.
2. A toothpick or larger object may be attached to dial so that participant need only grasp the protruding object to turn dial.
3. If participant has difficulty attending to one task, it may be helpful to cover all knobs, etc. except the intended one.
4. Homemade busy boxes can be constructed with the particular needs and abilities of the participant in mind, including lacing, buttoning, dialing, pushing buttons, sliding doors, etc.
5. There should be adequate space between the different components so that participant can attend to each individually.
6. Turning dial can be used as an excellent leadup skill for turning a telephone dial.
7. Dial may be replaced with larger dial and holes if participant is unable to place her finger in the small holes. Velcro strips or small magnets can also be used to aid the participant in grasping the dial in order to turn it.

CRAYONS

Name of Activity: Color Picture

Instructional Objective: Given a crayon and a picture from a coloring book of an apple, the participant will color the picture within the lines, 80% of the time.
Materials: crayon, table top, paper with outline of an apple on it
Verbal Cue: "Marsha, color the apple."

Task Analysis:
1. Pick up crayon and put in coloring position.
2. Extend nondominant arm downward toward paper, palm faced down.
3. Lower nondominant arm until palm makes contact with corresponding top corner of paper, holding it stationary.
4. Rotate wrist of dominant hand downward slightly, lowering point of crayon onto center of apple drawn on paper.
5. Scribble with crayon, staying within the lines of the apple picture.
6. Continue scribbling until entire apple has been colored inside the lines.

Activity Guidelines/Special Adaptations:
1. To help participant stay within the lines, a thick cardboard edge can be placed around external lines. This should only be used as necessary if participant has difficulty staying inside the lines. Use pictures with large areas to color, without irregular spaces.
2. Selection of colors should not be a prime concern initially, but only the use of a crayon within a confined area. It is best, therefore, to supply a limited number of crayons.

FRISBEE

Name of Activity: Throw Frisbee

Instructional Objective: Given a frisbee, the participant will throw the frisbee 5 feet, 80% of the time.
Materials: frisbee
Verbal Cue: "Kathy, throw the frisbee."

Task Analysis:
1. Extend dominant arm downward to frisbee, palm faced down.
2. Lower dominant arm until palm makes contact with edge of frisbee.
3. Curl fingers under frisbee.
4. Position thumb on top edge of frisbee.
5. Apply inward pressure between thumb and fingers to grasp frisbee firmly.

6. Bend elbow, raising frisbee to chest level, keeping it parallel to ground.
7. Raise dominant arm at shoulder, lifting frisbee to shoulder level.
8. Bend elbow, bringing frisbee inward toward chest.
9. Continue bending elbow until rim of frisbee makes contact with nondominant shoulder.
10. Quickly extend elbow outward away from body.
11. When elbow is fully extended, snap wrist outward 45°, simultaneously extending fingers, releasing frisbee in forward direction 1 foot.
12. Throw frisbee 2 feet.
13. Throw frisbee 3 feet.
14. Throw frisbee 4 feet.
15. Throw frisbee 5 feet.

Activity Guidelines/Special Adaptations:
1. Nerf frisbees that can be squeezed are available. This especially soft material will make the frisbee easier to hold.
2. If activity is done outdoors, a heavier frisbee can be used to overcome wind resistance.

Name of Activity: Catch Frisbee

Instructional Objective: Given a frisbee thrown by another person, the participant will catch the frisbee from 5 feet away, 80% of the time.
Materials: frisbee
Verbal Cue: "Kathy, catch the frisbee."

Task Analysis:
1. Stand 5 feet away from and facing other player, feet parallel and 6 inches apart.
2. Extend both arms outward toward other person, palms faced outward, fingers extended.
3. Follow path of frisbee through air.
4. As frisbee approaches, position palms directly parallel with frisbee.
5. When frisbee makes contact with palms, curl fingers inward toward palms until they are resting on top of frisbee, thumbs resting on underside of frisbee.
6. Apply inward pressure between fingers and thumbs to grasp frisbee firmly, catching frisbee.

Activity Guidelines/Special Adaptations:
1. Participant may practice catching the frisbee when it is slid across the floor to her; with proficiency, begin throwing frisbee through the air from a short distance, gradually increasing the distance from which it is thrown.

2. Some persons may find it easier to catch a larger frisbee, others may find a smaller frisbee easier to catch. Frisbees come in several sizes and weights and should be selected according to individual preference and skill level.
3. Initially, Nerf frisbee could be used to prevent injury and to make it easier to catch.

HANDGRIPPER

Name of Activity: Squeeze Handgripper

Instructional Objective: Given a handgripper, the participant will squeeze and release the handgripper 1 time with one hand, 80% of the time.
Materials: handgripper
Verbal Cue: "Larry, squeeze the handgripper."

Task Analysis:
1. Extend dominant arm downward toward handgripper (open end facing body), palm faced down.
2. Lower dominant arm until palm makes contact with handle.
3. Curl fingers around outer handle.
4. Wrap thumb around inner handle.
5. Apply inward pressure between thumb and fingers to grasp handle firmly.
6. Bend elbow, raising handgripper to chest level.
7. Apply steady inward pressure between thumb and fingers, squeezing handles toward each other.
8. Extend thumb and fingers slightly, allowing handles to return to original position.

Activity Guidelines/Special Adaptations:
1. This activity should be done with each hand in order to develop forearm strength equally.
2. Handgrippers are available with adjustable springs to suit the strength of the individual and to assure initial success.
3. Grippers may be used to help develop grasping skill in nondominant hand.
4. Participant can feel forearm muscle tense and relax as handgripper is squeezed and released, respectively.

HULA-HOOP

Name of Activity: Spin Hula-Hoop on Floor

Instructional Objective: Given a Hula-Hoop, the participant will spin the Hula-Hoop on the floor for 2 seconds, 50% of the time.

Materials: Hula-Hoop
Verbal Cue: "Georgia, spin the Hula-Hoop."

Task Analysis:
1. Stand facing hoop (held by another person), feet parallel and 6 inches apart.
2. Extend dominant arm outward toward top of Hula-Hoop, palm faced down.
3. Lower dominant arm until palm makes contact with top of hoop.
4. Curl fingers around top of hoop.
5. Wrap thumb around other side of hoop.
6. Apply inward pressure between thumb and fingers to grasp hoop firmly.
7. Extend elbow outward, bringing hoop to front of body, holding it 6 inches from and parallel to body.
8. Quickly rotate wrist upward and inward 90°, simultaneously extending fingers to release hoop, causing it to spin.
9. Spin Hula-Hoop for 1 second.
10. Spin Hula-Hoop for 2 seconds.

Activity Guidelines/Special Adaptations:
1. Participant may use fine motor skills to spin a top, ring, or small ball in a manner similar to spinning a hoop.
2. Floor surface should be smooth to allow for easier spinning motion of hoop, rather than attempting to spin hoop on a rug or a gravel surface.
3. Hoop may be wrapped with textured adhesive tape or sandpaper to give participant a better gripping surface at one particular spot.
4. A second person may support hoop while participant grips and spins it.

Name of Activity: Swing Hula-Hoop On Arm

Instructional Objective: Given a Hula-Hoop, the participant will swing the Hula-Hoop on her arm 2 consecutive times, 80% of the time.
Materials: Hula-Hoop
Verbal Cue: "Georgia, swing the Hula-Hoop on your arm."

Task Analysis:
1. Stand facing hoop (held by another person), feet parallel and 6 inches apart.
2. Extend nondominant arm outward toward top of Hula-Hoop, palm faced down.
3. Curl fingers around top of hoop.

4. Wrap thumb around other side of top of hoop.
5. Apply inward pressure between thumb and fingers to grasp hoop firmly.
6. Bend elbow of nondominant arm, raising hoop to chest level.
7. Extend dominant arm outward toward hoop, palm faced down.
8. Extend elbow of dominant arm until arm goes through center of hoop.
9. Extend fingers of nondominant hand, releasing hoop onto forearm of dominant arm.
10. Move nondominant arm downward toward side of body.
11. Rotate dominant arm clockwise in circular motion by pivoting arm at shoulder, causing hoop to swing on arm 1 time.
12. Swing Hula-Hoop on arm 2 times.

Activity Guidelines/Special Adaptations:
1. Merely holding up the hoop with the outstretched arm is an excellent exercise for strengthening the upper arm.
2. A small, lightweight hoop should be used initially. This will help the participant learn the proper arm motion with a minimum of resistance.
3. With proficiency, participant may transfer hoop from arm to arm while spinning it.
4. Participants may do this to music with a regular rhythmic pattern such as that of Hap Palmer.

Name of Activity: Twirl Hula-Hoop Around Waist

Instructional Objective: Given a Hula-Hoop, the participant will pick it up and twirl it around her waist 2 consecutive times, 50% of the time.

Materials: Hula-Hoop

Verbal Cue: "Georgia, twirl the Hula-Hoop around your waist."

Task Analysis:
1. Stand facing Hula-Hoop (lying on the floor), feet parallel and 6 inches apart.
2. Walk to Hula-Hoop.
3. Bend right knee, raising right foot 3 inches off ground.
4. Position right foot above center of hoop.
5. Extend right knee, lowering right foot to ground on inside of hoop.
6. Bend left knee, raising left foot 3 inches off ground.
7. Position left foot above center of hoop.
8. Extend left knee, lowering left foot to ground on inside of hoop.
9. Bend both knees, lowering body to ground.

10. Extend both arms outward toward opposite sides of hoop, palms faced down.
11. Lower both arms until palms make contact with each side of hoop.
12. Curl fingers around side of hoop.
13. Wrap thumbs around other side of hoop.
14. Apply inward pressure between thumb and fingers to grasp hoop firmly.
15. Extend both knees, raising body to standing position.
16. Extend both arms outward away from body until edge of hoop touches back of body at waist.
17. Move both arms 45° sideways at shoulders toward left side of body.
18. Quickly move both arms 45° sideways at shoulders toward right side of body, simultaneously extending fingers, releasing hoop.
19. Rotate hips in clockwise direction by moving knees and hips in clockwise circular direction, twirling Hula-Hoop around waist 1 time.
20. Twirl Hula-Hoop around waist second time.

Activity Guidelines/Special Adaptations:
1. A small hoop should initially be used in this activity since it will be easier to manipulate.
2. Participant may twirl to the beat of rhythmic music such as that of Hap Palmer.
3. Participant should push hoop in correct direction to give it momentum.

JACK-IN-THE-BOX

Name of Activity: Stuff Jack-in-the-Box

Instructional Objective: Given an open jack-in-the-box, the participant will stuff jack into the box, 80% of the time.

Materials: jack-in-the-box

Verbal Cue: "Robert, stuff jack into the box."

Task Analysis:
1. Extend dominant arm downward toward jack, palm faced down.
2. Lower dominant arm until palm makes contact with top of jack's head.
3. Extend elbow, apply downward pressure onto jack's head with palm.
4. Continue extending elbow, applying downward pressure until top of head is below base of lid.
5. Extend nondominant arm downward toward lid, palm faced down.
6. Lower nondominant arm until palm makes contact with top of lid.
7. Bend elbow of nondominant arm inward toward body, applying downward pressure onto lid with palm, lowering lid to box.

8. Continue bending elbow until lid makes contact with dominant hand holding jack's head down.
9. Move dominant arm sideways at shoulder, sliding hand out from under lid.
10. Extend elbow of nondominant arm, applying downward pressure onto lid.
11. Continue extending elbow until lid makes contact with box.
12. When click is heard, lid is secure and box has been closed.

Activity Guidelines/Special Adaptations:
1. If participant has use of only one hand, Dycem can be used under box so he can press clown down without sliding box. Box can also be held between legs while participant presses clown's head into box.
2. If participant has impaired use of hands, he can close lid using elbow, feet, or head pointer.
3. As clown's head is lowered, lid will move freely to closed position. When it is within 2 inches of being closed, direct pressure on top of lid will force head of clown down into box.

Name of Activity: Wind Jack-In-The-Box

Instructional Objective: Given a closed jack-in-the-box, the participant will wind the handle until jack pops out of the box, 80% of the time.
Materials: jack-in-the-box
Verbal Cue: "Robert, wind the jack-in-the-box."

Task Analysis:
1. Extend dominant hand downward toward handle, palm faced down, thumb and index finger extended.
2. Lower dominant arm until thumb and index finger make contact with each side of handle.
3. Apply inward pressure between thumb and index finger to grasp handle firmly.
4. Bend and extend elbow in a circular clockwise direction, rotating handle clockwise.
5. Continue winding handle until jack pops out of box.

Activity Guidelines/Special Adaptations:
1. Participant may need to use other fingers or palm to wind handle.
2. Handle may be enlarged by wrapping it with sponge and tape to allow for easier manipulation. Handle can also be extended by attaching wooden dowel to it.
3. Have participant say, "Pop goes the weasel!" when jack's head pops out of box.

MARBLES

Name of Activity: Roll Marble

Instructional Objective: Given a marble, the participant will pick up the marble without dropping it, and roll it at least 1 foot toward the target area, 80% of the time.
Materials: large marble
Verbal Cue: "Jimmy, pick up the marble."

Task Analysis:
1. Extend dominant arm downward toward marble, palm faced down, thumb and index finger extended.
2. Lower dominant arm until thumb and index finger make contact with opposite sides of marble.
3. Apply inward pressure between thumb and index finger to grasp marble firmly.
4. Bend elbow, lifting marble to chest level.
5. Stand 1 foot away from and facing target area, feet parallel and 6 inches apart.
6. Bend knees, lowering body toward ground.
7. Lower knees to ground.
8. Bend forward at waist 45°.
9. Extend dominant arm holding marble downward toward ground.
10. Position dominant hand holding marble 6 inches to the side of dominant knee, elbow fully extended, palm facing forward.
11. Bring dominant hand backward 6 inches, keeping elbow fully extended.
12. Swing dominant arm forward 12 inches, simultaneously extending fingers, releasing marble, rolling it toward target area.
13. Roll marble 4 inches.
14. Roll marble 6 inches.
15. Roll marble 8 inches.
16. Roll marble 1 foot.

Activity Guidelines/Special Adaptations:
1. A jumbo size marble can be used initially; with proficiency, progress to smaller marbles.
2. If participant has a tendency to put objects in his mouth, it may be advisable not to use marbles. In any case, activities using marbles should be strictly supervised.
3. If participant is unable to pick up marbles individually, a scoop may be held or attached to hand for use in picking them up.
4. Various targets can be used: a coffee can, a person, a shoe box, etc. The purpose is to give direction to the roll. Initially, target should be

large enough and close enough to participant to ensure initial success. With proficiency, reduce size of target area and increase distance.
5. If participant is unable to grasp the marble, he may roll it with hand or foot.
6. Rolling marbles in a confined area is a good idea so that marbles do not scatter and become a hazard. A corner of a room would be a good location.

Name of Activity: Shoot Marble

Instructional Objective: Given a large marble, the participant will shoot the marble with his thumb 1 foot to the target area, 80% of the time.
Materials: large marble
Verbal Cue: "Jimmy, shoot the marble."

Task Analysis:
1. Pick up marble.
2. Stand 1 foot away from and facing target area, feet parallel and 6 inches apart.
3. Bend knees, lowering body toward ground.
4. Lower knees to ground.
5. Bend forward at waist 45°.
6. Extend dominant arm holding marble downward toward ground, 3 inches in front of dominant knee, palm facing inward.
7. Lower dominant arm until hand makes contact with ground.
8. Bend index finger, circling it around marble, cradling marble in finger.
9. Position thumb directly behind marble, thumbnail touching marble.
10. Quickly extend thumb forward, applying forward pressure onto marble with thumb, causing marble to shoot forward toward target area.
11. Shoot marble 4 inches.
12. Shoot marble 6 inches.
13. Shoot marble 8 inches.
14. Shoot marble 1 foot.

Activity Guidelines/Special Adaptations:
1. Target should initially be a large area and with proficiency become smaller.
2. If participant lacks fine motor control to shoot marbles, he can simply roll them or push them toward the target area.
3. A large game of marbles can be designed using foam rubber Nerf balls rather than marbles, and using a much larger circle. This may

be especially useful for participants lacking fine motor control necessary to shoot marbles.

MR. BUBBLE

Name of Activity: Open Bottle

Instructional Objective: Given a bottle of Mr. Bubble, the participant will unscrew the top and remove it, without spilling any liquid, 80% of the time.
Materials: Mr. Bubble
Verbal Cue: "Gary, open the bottle."

Task Analysis:
1. Extend nondominant arm forward toward bottle, hand slightly cupped, thumb closest to and parallel with body.
2. Curl fingers and thumb around opposite sides of bottle.
3. Apply inward pressure between thumb and fingers to grasp bottle firmly.
4. Bend elbow, raising bottle to chest level.
5. Extend dominant arm upward toward lid of bottle, palm faced down, hand slightly cupped.
6. Lower dominant arm until palm makes contact with lid.
7. Curl fingers around one side of lid.
8. Wrap thumb around other side of lid.
9. Apply inward pressure between thumb and fingers to grasp lid firmly.
10. Rotate wrist of dominant hand counterclockwise, simultaneously rotating wrist of nondominant hand clockwise.
11. Extend fingers of dominant hand, releasing grasp on lid.
12. Unscrew lid of bottle further.
13. Raise dominant arm upward at shoulder, lifting lid off bottle.

Activity Guidelines/Special Adaptations:
1. Commercial jar lid openers are available that will hold the lid of the container stationary so that participant can turn the container with one hand to open jar. A piece of Dycem can be placed under jar to hold it in place for participants with use of only one hand.
2. Rough-textured adhesive tape or sandpaper can be applied to edges of lid to provide a better gripping surface. A larger lid can also be applied to original lid if participant has difficulty grasping a smaller one.
3. Teacher may loosen the lid initially to aid in removal and to ensure success for participant.

4. While blowing bubbles may be reinforcing for many participants, a jar containing edibles may be more motivating.

Name of Activity: Blow Bubble

Instructional Objective: Given a bottle of Mr. Bubble, the participant will remove the wand from the bottle and blow 1 bubble from the wand, 80% of the time.
Materials: Mr. Bubble, wand
Verbal Cue: "Gary, blow a bubble."

Task Analysis:
1. Remove Mr. Bubble top.
2. Remove wand from bottle.
3. Bend elbow of dominant arm, slowly bringing the wand upward to mouth level.
4. Position circular end of wand containing Mr. Bubble liquid 2 inches from and parallel to mouth.
5. Gently inhale through mouth.
6. Gently blow air into the wand until a bubble is formed and is released from the wand.

Activity Guidelines/Special Adaptations:
1. This activity may serve as a leadup activity to blowing bubbles with bubble gum, which requires more sustained breath control.
2. The wand should initially be held close to mouth to ensure success. With proficiency, the participant can hold it further away, requiring a more sustained burst of air.
3. This activity can be used to develop better breath control which is important in good speech production as well as stamina in physical activities.

MULTIPURPOSE BALL

Name of Activity: Roll Ball

Instructional Objective: Given a multipurpose ball, the participant will roll the ball 10 feet, 80% of the time.
Materials: multipurpose ball
Verbal Cue: "Cary, roll the ball."

Task Analysis:
1. Stand directly behind ball, feet parallel and 6 inches apart.
2. Bend knees, lowering body toward ground.

3. Bend at waist 45°.
4. Extend elbows, bringing arms downward to sides of ball, palms faced inward.
5. Move arms inward at shoulder until palms make contact with opposite sides of ball.
6. Apply inward pressure between palms to grasp ball firmly.
7. Bend elbows, raising ball to chest level.
8. Extend elbows quickly, moving arms forward away from body, simultaneously extending fingers, releasing ball onto ground and rolling it forward 4 feet.
9. Roll ball 6 feet.
10. Roll ball 8 feet.
11. Roll ball 10 feet.

Activity Guidelines/Special Adaptations:
1. This activity can be played as a roly poly game, having participant and other player (or teacher) sit with legs extended and bottoms of feet positioned against each other. The ball is then rolled to other player with legs acting as boundaries.
2. Ball can be rolled off a chair with participant sitting in the chair. A ball that is pushed or hit off the chair will subsequently bounce and roll in the anticipated direction.
3. If participant cannot extend arms to push the ball, a small incline can initially be used. The participant only has to release the ball on top of the incline and ball will roll down.
4. When choosing a ball, bear in mind the variety in size, texture, and color.

Name of Activity: Kick Ball

Instructional Objective: Given a multipurpose ball, the participant will kick the ball 10 feet, 80% of the time.
Materials: multipurpose ball
Verbal Cue: "Cary, kick the ball."

Task Analysis:
1. Stand directly behind ball, feet parallel and 6 inches apart.
2. Bend knee of dominant leg, bringing foot backward behind body (all weight is now on nondominant leg).
3. Extend knee of dominant leg, bringing foot forward toward ball with toes pointing toward ball.
4. Continue forward motion of foot until toes make contact with ball, kicking ball forward 4 feet.
5. Kick ball forward 6 feet.

6. Kick ball forward 8 feet.
7. Kick ball forward 10 feet.

Activity Guidelines/Special Adaptations:
1. Once kicking a stationary ball has been mastered, the participant can attempt to kick a ball that is rolled to him. This skill is used in more complex games such as kickball and soccer.
2. Kicking a ball can be taught while the participant is sitting in a chair with legs hanging down to the floor. This enables participant to kick a ball without having to balance on the nondominant foot.

Name of Activity: Throw Ball

Instructional Objective: Given a multipurpose ball, the participant will throw the ball 10 feet through the air, 80% of the time.
Materials: multipurpose ball
Verbal Cue: "Cary, throw the ball."

Task Analysis:
1. Stand directly behind ball, feet parallel and 6 inches apart.
2. Bend knees, lowering rear toward ground.
3. Bend at waist 45°.
4. Extend both arms outward toward ball, palms faced inward.
5. Move arms inward at shoulder until palms make contact with sides of ball.
6. Apply inward pressure between palms to grasp ball firmly.
7. Bend elbows, raising ball to chest level.
8. Extend knees, raising body to upright position.
9. Extend elbows fully, bringing arms outward away from body.
10. Raise arms upward at shoulder 90°, bringing ball above head.
11. Bend elbows 45°, bringing ball behind head.
12. Quickly extend elbows 90°, bringing hands and forearms forward over head, simultaneously extending fingers, releasing ball into air 4 feet.
13. Throw ball 6 feet.
14. Throw ball 8 feet.
15. Throw ball 10 feet.

Activity Guidelines/Special Adaptations:
1. A heavy ball is easier for the ataxic and the athetoid person to play with, because their movements are so disorganized and clumsy that a standard ball may roll away. A spastic child, on the other hand, can play best with a smaller solid ball, because his grip may be too firm and he will have difficulty lifting a heavy ball. A hemiplegic child

should play with a large beach ball to encourage him to use both hands together.

SCISSORS

Name of Activity: Open and Close Scissors (Cutting Movement)

Instructional Objective: Given a pair of scissors, the participant will open and close the scissors 3 consecutive times, 80% of the time.
Materials: 4-inch blunt end scissors
Verbal Cue: "Donna, open and close the scissors."

Task Analysis:
1. Extend dominant arm downward toward handle of scissors.
2. Spread and extend thumb and index finger of dominant hand.
3. Position thumb and index finger above holes in scissors handle.
4. Pass thumb and index finger through finger holes.
5. Bend index finger downward against lower edge of top hole.
6. Apply inward pressure between thumb and index finger to grasp scissors firmly.
7. Bend elbow, raising scissors to chest level.
8. Rotate wrist 90° clockwise until palm is facing inward, thumb on top (handshake position).
9. Extend scissors outward away from body by extending elbow.
10. Extend thumb, raising it as far as it will go, moving top hole of scissors handle away from index finger.
11. Lower thumb to index finger to close scissors.
12. Open scissors second time.
13. Close scissors second time.
14. Open scissors third time.
15. Close scissors third time.

Activity Guidelines/Special Adaptations:
1. Training scissors are available with four finger holes that allow for both the participant and the teacher to grasp the scissors and cut together. This allows the participant to experience the scissor movement even though unable to manipulate independently.
2. The sharpness of the point and the size of the scissors may vary with available resources. Just as it is important not to expose participants to unnecessary danger, it is also important not to give them scissors with edges that are too blunt and that require great effort to operate. Participants should be able to experience success with reasonable effort.
3. Special education scissors are also available for those with eye-hand

coordination difficulties. Polypropylene handles can be squeezed together by hands, arms, or other body part.

Name of Activity: Cut Paper on Straight Line

Instructional Objective: Given a pair of scissors and a piece of paper, the participant will cut a 5-inch straight line, staying within 1/4 inch of either side of the line, 80% of the time.
Materials: 4-inch blunt end scissors, paper with 5-inch line
Verbal Cue: "Donna, cut the paper on the line."

Task Analysis:
1. Hold scissors in cutting position in dominant hand, at chest level.
2. Extend nondominant hand downward toward corner of paper.
3. Curl tip of index finger under one corner of paper.
4. Place thumb on top of same corner of paper.
5. Apply inward finger pressure to grasp paper firmly.
6. Lift paper to chest level by bending at elbow.
7. Raise dominant thumb as far as it will spread from index finger to open scissors.
8. Place inner opening of blade of scissors against near edge of paper on end of line by extending elbow.
9. Lower thumb to index finger to cut line 1 inch.
10. Cut line 2 inches.
11. Cut line 3 inches.
12. Cut line 4 inches.
13. Cut line 5 inches.

Activity Guidelines/Special Adaptations:
1. Line should be drawn on paper with a color that sharply contrasts with paper. A 1/4-inch margin should be left on either side of the line with cardboard borders along the outer edges of the margins that the participant cannot cut through.
2. If participant has difficulty holding scissors and paper at the same time, teacher may hold paper stationary, allowing participant to concentrate exclusively on manipulation of the scissors.

Name of Activity: Cut Out Picture

Instructional Objective: Given a pair of scissors and a picture of an apple, the participant will cut the apple out of the paper, staying within 1/4 inch of either side of the picture, 80% of the time.
Materials: 4-inch blunt end scissors, magazine picture
Verbal Cue: "Donna, cut out the picture."

Task Analysis:
1. Hold scissors in cutting position in dominant hand at chest level.
2. Hold paper firmly in nondominant hand at chest level.
3. Cut outer line of picture until curve is reached.
4. Raise thumb to open scissors.
5. Keeping scissors open and stationary, rotate wrist of nondominant hand to turn paper so that scissors are always aligned with outer line of picture.
6. Continue cutting until entire picture is cut out.

Activity Guidelines/Special Adaptations:
1. This skill can be implemented in conjunction with scrapbook activities. Participant will be most attentive if really interested in saving the picture she is cutting out.
2. Initially, there should be a distinct cutting line with sharp contrast to the areas on either side of the lines. A broad marking pen can be used to emphasize the cutting line. Pictures should initially consist of straight lines and simple curves.
3. With proficiency, allow participants to scan magazines and select their own pictures to be cut out. This may be more effective if colorfully illustrated magazines are used.

SLINKY

Name of Activity: Stretch Slinky

Instructional Objective: Given a Slinky, the participant will stretch the Slinky from a compressed form to a length of 1 foot without dropping it, 80% of the time.
Materials: Slinky
Verbal Cue: "Scott, stretch the Slinky."

Task Analysis:
1. Extend both arms downward toward ends of Slinky, palms faced inward, fingers spread apart.
2. Lower arms until palms make contact with open ends of Slinky.
3. Curl fingers around outer edges of Slinky.
4. Wrap thumbs around opposite sides of edges of Slinky.
5. Apply inward pressure between thumbs and fingers to grasp Slinky firmly.
6. Bend elbows, raising Slinky to chest level.
7. Move arms outward at shoulders, moving hands toward opposite sides of body, stretching Slinky 4 inches.

8. Stretch Slinky 6 inches.
9. Stretch Slinky 8 inches.
10. Stretch Slinky 1 foot.

Activity Guidelines/Special Adaptations:
1. Wrap exposed ends of Slinky with adhesive tape to prevent participant from poking himself with the loose ends.
2. A standard size Slinky may be cumbersome for the participant. If so, smaller sized Slinkys are available and may be substituted.
3. This activity can be done by supporting the Slinky on a lapboard or table and stretching the ends. If participant has use of only one hand, one end of Slinky can be held stationary between the legs and the other end stretched upward with the hand. This activity can be used as a leadup activity to isometric exercises and lifting dumbbells.

Name of Activity: Walk Slinky Down Steps

Instructional Objective: Given a Slinky, the participant will position the Slinky on the top of 3 steps and cause it to "walk" down the steps to the bottom, 80% of the time.
Materials: Slinky, steps
Verbal Cue: "Scott, walk the Slinky down the steps."

Task Analysis:
1. Extend both arms downward toward open ends of Slinky, palms faced inward, fingers spread apart.
2. Lower arms until palms make contact with ends of Slinky.
3. Curl fingers around one side of edges of Slinky.
4. Wrap thumbs around opposite sides of edges of Slinky.
5. Apply inward pressure between thumbs and fingers to grasp Slinky firmly.
6. Bend elbows, raising Slinky to chest level.
7. Walk to stairs.
8. Bend knees, lowering body toward ground.
9. Position dominant hand near edge of top step.
10. Lower dominant arm until edge of Slinky makes contact with edge of first step.
11. Lower nondominant arm until opposite edge of Slinky makes contact with center of second step.
12. Extend fingers of dominant hand, releasing top of Slinky, causing it to "walk" to second step.
13. Extend fingers of nondominant hand, releasing Slinky, causing it to "walk" to bottom step.

Activity Guidelines/Special Adaptations:
1. This activity should be done on a small set of stairs initially, especially if participant has any problems with balance. With proficiency, and supervision, the participant can do this on a larger set of steps.
2. Uncarpeted sets will facilitate the most regular movement of the Slinky down the stairs. Steps may be fashioned out of cardboard boxes if it is not feasible to use a set of stairs.

TELEPHONE

Name of Activity: Answer Telephone

Instructional Objective: Given a table telephone that is ringing, the participant will pick up the receiver before the fifth ring and begin conversation with appropriate greeting, 100% of the time.
Materials: telephone
Verbal Cue: "Mark, answer the telephone."

Task Analysis:
1. Bend knees, lowering body to chair, assuming sitting position, arm's reach from telephone.
2. Extend dominant arm outward toward receiver, palm faced down.
3. Position hand directly above center of receiver.
4. Lower dominant arm until palm makes contact with receiver (mouthpiece facing pinky).
5. Curl fingers around receiver.
6. Wrap thumb around other side of receiver.
7. Apply inward pressure between thumb and fingers to grasp receiver firmly.
8. Raise arm at shoulder, lifting receiver up off telephone.
9. Bend elbow, raising receiver to head level on dominant side of body.
10. Rotate wrist clockwise until palm and earphone face nondominant side of body.
11. Raise elbow to lift earphone to ear level.
12. Place earphone onto ear by moving dominant arm further inward toward nondominant side of body.
13. While holding earphone to ear, rotate wrist in proper direction to align mouthpiece with mouth.
14. Say, "Hello, this is (name), may I help you?"
15. Await response from caller.

Activity Guidelines/Special Adaptations:
1. If participant has a noticeable hearing loss in one ear, teacher should make sure that the earphone of the receiver is placed against the more

efficient ear. In such cases, the dominant hand may not necessarily be used.
2. Painting or taping a picture of a mouth on the mouthpiece and an ear on the earpiece will allow the participant to match the pictures to his own body parts and to distinguish the different functions of each end of the receiver, thereby facilitating proper positioning of the phone.
3. A tape recorder may be used to record and play back the participant's initial greeting on the telephone. Inexpensive walkie-talkies, as well as wrist radios, can also be utilized.
4. Many individuals choose to pick up the receiver in their nondominant hand, freeing their dominant hand for dialing the telephone. Others may need to lift the receiver with their dominant hand.

Name of Activity: Deposit Money In Pay Telephone

Instructional Objective: Given a pay telephone and the correct change (20 cents) in participant's pocket, the participant will take the change out of his pocket, pick up the receiver, and place the coins into the coin slot, 80% of the time.

Materials: pay telephone, exact change for call (e.g., 2 dimes)
Verbal Cue: "Mark, put the money into the telephone."

Task Analysis:
1. Enter telephone station.
2. Raise dominant hand above participant's pocket by raising elbow, palm faced inward.
3. Lower hand into pocket by lowering elbow and extending arm downward.
4. Curl 4 fingers around dimes.
5. Continue to curl fingers until coins are surrounded by fingers in palm.
6. Lift hand from pants pocket by raising elbow.
7. Extend arm outward toward phone book shelf, palm faced down.
8. Position fist over phone book shelf.
9. Lower hand to shelf by lowering arm at shoulder.
10. Extend fingers, releasing coins onto shelf.
11. Lift receiver.
12. Listen for dial tone (when dial tone is heard, continue).
13. Point index finger and thumb of dominant hand toward first dime by extending two fingers.
14. Lower fingers to first dime by extending elbow.
15. Continue to lower hand until index finger makes contact with coin.
16. Curl nail of index finger around and underneath outer edge of coin.

17. Place tip of thumb on opposite side of coin.
18. Apply inward pressure between thumb and finger to grasp coin firmly.
19. Raise hand holding coin upward to coin slot by extending at elbow.
20. Rotate wrist toward dominant side of body to align coin with coin slot.
21. Rotate wrist outward toward coin slot, forcing coin into slot.
22. Force tip of thumb against coin slot by bending thumb at second joint.
23. Listen for coin to fall.
24. Deposit second dime into coin slot.
25. Listen for second dime to fall and for dial tone.

Activity Guidelines/Special Adaptations:
1. Coin and coin slot can be color-coded to aid participant in matching the proper coin and coin slot initially. Begin by using a single coin rather than mixing nickels and dimes.
2. Rather than using an actual pay telephone and investing several dimes, a small cardboard box can be arranged alongside a home telephone with appropriate slots cut out for either coins, pokerchips, or cardboard tokens.
3. Placing money in a piggy bank or similar home bank can be used as a leadup activity to placing coins in the telephone.
4. All telephone areas for public use must contain at least one telephone that can be used by the physically disabled, including people in wheelchairs and those with hearing and sight disabilities. Telephone booths should be avoided; use the open type telephone station.
5. According to the Virginia Commission of Outdoor Recreation, telephone booths and telephones must meet the following requirements: a) telephone booths must have a 32-inch clear entrance; b) telephones must be placed so that dial, receiver, and coin drop are no more than 4 feet above the floor.
6. If participant cannot take change out of his pants pocket, place coins on top of phone book shelf, allowing participant to pick the coins up and deposit them into phone.

Name of Activity: Dial Phone Number

Instructional Objective: Given a telephone and a specified 7-digit number, the participant will dial the phone number and listen for the party to answer, or for a busy signal, 80% of the time.
Materials: telephone
Verbal Cue: "Mark, dial the number."

Task Analysis:
1. Enter telephone station.
2. Lift receiver in nondominant hand.
3. Deposit money in pay telephone with dominant hand.
4. Listen for coins to drop and for dial tone.
5. Extend dominant arm outward toward telephone dial, palm faced down, index finger extended.
6. Extend elbow, moving hand forward toward first digit of number.
7. Rotate wrist in clockwise direction until index finger reaches fingerstop.
8. Bend elbow, removing index finger from digit hole.
9. Observe telephone dial rotating counterclockwise to original position.
10. Dial second digit with index finger.
11. Dial third digit.
12. Dial fourth digit.
13. Dial fifth digit.
14. Dial sixth digit.
15. Dial seventh digit.
16. Observe telephone dial rotating counterclockwise to original position.
17. Listen for party to answer or for busy signal.
18. If busy signal is heard, extend nondominant arm, holding receiver, outward to telephone.
19. Rotate wrist outward until earpiece faces telephone receiver holder.
20. Position earpiece directly above holder.
21. Lower arm at shoulder, placing receiver onto holder, hanging up the phone.
22. Extend fingers, releasing receiver onto holder.
23. If party answers, speak with person.

Activity Guidelines/Special Adaptations:
1. While it would be a useful, long-term skill to be able to dial designated phone numbers, this can also serve as a valuable exercise in developing eye-hand and fine motor coordination.
2. Since the numbers and letters of the dial may offer little meaning to the participant, it may be helpful to place different colored circles on top of the digits and letters, and to use this to practice color discrimination.
3. There are play phones available that will "talk" or play music when a certain number or picture is dialed; there are usually several different programs on each phone. This would serve as a reinforcement for appropriate dialing behavior.
4. There are dial toys available that can be used in a leadup activity to

dialing the telephone. One of the toys involves a picture of an animal; the sound that the animal makes is played when that picture is dialed. This can be reinforcing for the participant.
5. Pushbutton telephones may be used to eliminate the need to dial the phone.
6. A classroom kit entitled "How to Use the Telephone (The Dial-a-Phone Kit)" published by the Instructo Corporation and written by Ruth Leff is presently available. The kit has been field-tested with trainable mentally retarded children and adults and individuals in learning disability classes. It includes a phonograph record of telephone signals and an actual call to operator, number sequence slides, a number color dial, and telephone reminder posters for several individuals.
7. Have participants practice dialing phone numbers by posting the number of the weather or time on a board and allowing them to call the numbers and listen to the reports.

Name of Activity: Talk On Telephone

Instructional Objective: Given a telephone and a friend's phone number that has already been dialed, the participant will talk on the telephone with the answering party for at least 10 seconds and then hang up the phone, 100% of the time.

Materials: telephone

Verbal Cue: "Mark, talk on the phone."

Task Analysis:
1. Listen for person to answer phone.
2. Respond by saying, "Hello, this is (name). How are you, (answering party's name)?"
3. Listen for response to question (e.g., "I am fine, (caller's name), and how are you doing?").
4. Respond by saying, "I am fine, thank you."
5. Continue conversation by stating purpose of call (e.g., "Would you like to go to the movies today?").
6. Listen for response to question (e.g., "Yes, I would like to go.").
7. Respond with time of day to meet.
8. End conversation with appropriate farewell (e.g., "I will see you at 7 o'clock. Good-bye.").
9. Listen for response (e.g., "Bye-bye.").
10. After 10 seconds of conversation, extend nondominant arm holding receiver outward toward telephone.
11. Rotate wrist outward until earpiece faces telephone receiver holder.

12. Position earpiece directly above holder.
13. Lower arm at shoulder, placing receiver onto holder, hanging up phone.
14. Extend elbow, allowing arm to fall to side.

Activity Guidelines/Special Adaptations:
1. In cases where the participant is reluctant to initiate a phone conversation, there are play telephones available that will "talk" to the participant when dialed; this provides an excellent way to prompt the participant to answer specific questions. The phone usually has several different programs such as "How are you?", "What is your name?", etc.
2. Accomplishment cards are available from the Bell Telephone System that verify that the card holder has exhibited competence in the utilization of a telephone. This may help to reinforce participant's feeling of success.
3. If the participant is unable to hold the receiver up to his ear and mouth, a device is available that enables the participant to rest the receiver on his shoulder, aligning his ear and mouth with the receiver's components.
4. Receivers can be equipped with an adjustable audio control device that can increase the sound level of those with hearing deficiencies.
5. A good and inexpensive way to practice talking on the phone is by joining together two hollow cardboard cylinders with a piece of string, making a makeshift phone. If you cover one end with waxed paper, you will find that the sounds will be amplified and the participants can speak to one another from a distance.
6. Excellent role playing exercises can be performed, having participants take part in various conversations and situations (e.g., calling fire department during an emergency).
7. It would also be appropriate for nonverbal individuals to learn to pick up the receiver, dial, and deposit coins into a telephone. We feel that it is not essential to be able to verbalize to learn to manipulate a telephone.

VENDING MACHINE

Name of Activity: Use of Vending Machine

Instructional Objective: Given a vending machine and money, the participant will place the proper amount of change into the coin slot and pull the lever of a selected item, 80% of the time.

Materials: vending machine, money
Verbal Cue: "Toby, use the vending machine."

Task Analysis:
1. Select item to be purchased.
2. Extend dominant hand holding coin outward toward coin slot.
3. Position edge of coin directly in front of coin slot.
4. Push coin into coin slot by extending at elbow.
5. Listen for coin to drop.
6. Place index finger of dominant hand on button of selected item.
7. Push button by extending index finger and applying forward pressure onto button with finger.
8. Release button by withdrawing hand from machine.
9. Extend dominant hand into produce access slot.
10. Grasp item in access slot with dominant hand using palmar grasp.
11. Take item out of machine by withdrawing hand.

Activity Guidelines/Special Adaptations:
1. If a vending machine is not easily accessible for practice, one can be constructed from cardboard for instructional purposes. Poker chips or round pieces of cardboard (same size as coins) can be used as money.
2. The use of pictures, along with the brand name logo, can be used to aid participant in discerning the items contained in the vending machine.
3. Initially, participant should be given exact change so that he does not have to select change. Eventually, elementary monetary concepts can be introduced in conjunction with this activity; participant can learn to place the proper amount of money into the machine to obtain desired item or will learn to expect change in the change slot.
4. Most vending machines now use push buttons rather than levers; however, it would be a good idea to incorporate machines with levers into this activity since the participant will probably encounter levers at some time.
5. Participant can be encouraged to ask for assistance from a nonhandicapped bystander, particularly if he has motor difficulties. Nonverbal participants can practice showing money to bystander while simultaneously pointing to desired item—this will communicate a request for assistance.
6. It is a widely recognized fact of life that machines do not always respond as expected; therefore, it is important to teach participants the function of the coin return. Also, teaching the participants to try

the machine several times is important, because the coins are not always properly "digested" on the first attempt. Ultimately, however, the participant should be prepared for the disappointment that occurs when he is robbed of not only the opportunity to obtain a desired item, but also of his money.

Chapter 10
PROGRAM IMPLEMENTATION
Illustrations of Recreational Competence

To this point, information has been presented concerning the philosophical basis of this text, normalization theory. Assessment and skill selection techniques, material and skill adaptations, and instructional guidelines for program development were also presented in subsequent chapters. Following these guidelines, an extensive task analytic-based curriculum was presented in the skill areas of hobbies, sports, games, and object manipulation.

To fully understand the previously presented material and how it relates to a coherently implemented program, it is necessary to describe data-based programs that feature successful change in leisure behavior of clients. Therefore, this chapter is devoted exclusively to discussing several behavioral programs implemented for the purpose of developing and generalizing leisure skills in disabled clients. We have purposely focused on the more severely handicapped population. An effort has also been made to feature chronologically age-appropriate leisure skills for instruction with the adolescent and adult population. Daily collection of data on each of the programs implemented provided assessment data relevant to the degree of skill generalization exhibited by the participant(s).

CASE STUDY I: TEACHING THE USE OF A CAMERA TO A MULTIPLY HANDICAPPED WOMAN

In order to help handicapped individuals learn to independently recreate with chronolgoical age-appropriate activities, two categories of trainer intervention can be identified. First, *instructional techniques* may be employed. Second, *programmatic adaptations* of leisure activities may be considered as a viable option for increasing participation, especially in those individuals with severe physical or sensory impairments. The case below emphasizes the successful interaction of these interventions by teaching a multiply handicapped woman the independent use of a camera.

Participant and Setting

Ruth is 23 years old and severely handicapped. She is paralyzed from the waist down and confined to a wheelchair. Due to her spina bifida and hydrocephaly, Ruth has difficulty holding her head erect. Tremors are prevalent as she moves her arms away from midline. Her arm movement is limited because of stiffness at her elbows. Ruth's IQ score is in the mild retardation range. She has a history of seizures that are currently being controlled through the use of dilantin and phenobarbitol. One major problem regarding her potential for independent living reported by parents and staff is her reluctance to initiate activities. This also extends to her self-care maintenance program. Ruth requires constant prompting to complete the majority of her basic tasks. She has not been moved to a sheltered workshop due to her significantly low rates of work production. Ruth's AAMD Adaptive Behavior Scale scores include a significant degree of withdrawal, as well as significantly poor independent functioning and physical development. She is currently attending an adult developmental center that offers self-help, social/communication, and prevocational skills training to 12 severely and profoundly handicapped persons between 21 and 63 years of age. A bus picks the clients up daily at 9 a.m. at their homes and transports them to and from the center, returning home at 3 p.m. Leisure skills training takes place in the recreation room within the center. This room contains leisure-related materials and equipment.

Program Objective

The objective of the leisure skills training was to teach Ruth to take photographs using a One-Step Polaroid Camera. To reach criterion, Ruth had to place the neck strap over her head, lift the camera to eye level, center the subject in the viewfinder, and take the photograph of the candidate whom she had previously asked to pose. Finally, Ruth had to remove the photograph from the camera and watch it develop. The candidate being photographed had to appear in the picture, and this photography skill had to be accomplished 100% of the time with only a verbal cue being given.

A secondary objective was to generalize the photography skill to four other environments and to initiate picture taking without the verbal cue 80% of the time.

The rationale for selection of this activity was because a) Ruth expressed an interest in learning this skill; b) parents expressed interest in this hobby via a parent recreational interest inventory; c) it is age-appropriate; d) it facilitates social interaction with handicapped and nonhandicapped peers; e) it provides immediate reinforcement with a photograph in 60 seconds; and f) the skill requires manipulation of the camera at midline, which is commensurate with Ruth's physical abilities.

Procedure

Instructional sessions were conducted 5 days per week, 15 minutes per session. Sessions were held at different times during the day, between 9:30 a.m. and noon. Instruction was performed at different times in order to facilitate generalization of the skill.

An 11-step task analysis was utilized to identify the component subskills of this complex task. The component steps consisted of: a) requesting permission of candidate being photographed; b) positioning camera; c) manipulation of shutter release button; and d) removing photograph from camera. These component steps were in turn categorized into the 11 task-analyzed steps. The task analysis was acquired from earlier curriculum work.

To obtain content validity, several persons owning a One-Step Polaroid Camera were asked to review the necessary responses required to operate it. See Table 1 for a task analysis of the use of a One-Step Polaroid Camera.

Initial baseline data were taken during five consecutive days with one session per day. The general verbal cue, "Ruth, take a picture of (name of person being photographed)," was given, and the response recorded.

Following initial baseline, the trainer determined which step instruc-

Table 1. Use of a One-step Polaroid camera

Verbal Cue: "Ruth, take a picture of (another individual's name)."

1. Ask other individual, "Can I take a picture of you?"
2. If reply is "*Yes*", point to where individual should sit/stand (Not more than 12 feet away).
3. Ask individual to smile/wave.
4. Grasp opposite sides of camera with both hands using palmar grasps (Lens facing away from body).
5. Bend arms at elbows to raise camera to eye level until viewfinder is 1 inch in front of dominant eye.
6. Center other individual in viewfinder to complete preparation for picture taking.
7. Extend index finger of dominant hand and position directly in front of shutter release button.
8. Bend index finger at second joint, applying pressure onto button, pushing button in until completely depressed.
9. Wait for photograph to descend from camera base.
10. Remove photograph from camera.
11. Attend to photograph for 5 seconds.

tion was to begin. If a step was performed successfully on two consecutive trials, instruction would begin on the following step of the sequence. Each of the two consecutive trials on the step must have been performed within 15 seconds of the verbal cue and without additional prompting provided. Additionally, the participant had to reach criterion on all preceding steps.

Instruction began on the sixth session utilizing a three step cue hierarchy ranging from least to most instrusive (Sulzer-Azaroff & Mayer, 1977). The trainer first provided the verbal cue and praise was provided for a correct response. An incorrect response led to the second step of the cue hierarchy. The trainer repeated the verbal cue and guided the appropriate response. Praise was then provided for a correct behavior. Another incorrect response led to the third step of the hierarchy. The trainer once again gave the verbal cue and physically guided the participant through the behavior.

Five training trials on one step were performed each session. Following the trials, the general verbal cue was given and the responses recorded. No modeling or physical prompting were offered during this final nonreinforced probe. Criterion for mastery of the entire skill was reached after the participant successfully performed all steps of the task analysis for five consecutive sessions (100% of the time).

Special Adaptations

A special material adaptation was used during the program to simplify the activity. A 1/2-inch piece of wax crayon was attached to the shutter release button following several unsuccessful attempts to depress the button during initial balance. It was agreed upon by all staff and participant that the appropriate manipulation of the camera would be an impossible task without the adaptation. At that time, baseline and subsequent training commenced utilizing the modified equipment. Figure 1 provides an illustration of the adapted camera.

A modification of the skill sequence was also introduced. An initial task analysis was developed based on a normal individual's performance on the skill. However, because of Ruth's poor fine motor functioning, the step requiring her to position her index finger over the shutter release button had to be taught before she raised the camera to eye level. In this fashion, Ruth was able to center the subject in the viewfinder and immediately take the photograph, while maintaining control of the camera. Additionally, this adaptation eliminated the need to search for the shutter release button which previously had been difficult.

Generalization

In order to verify the generalization of the camera skill in other more relevant environments, generalization probes were taken in four other

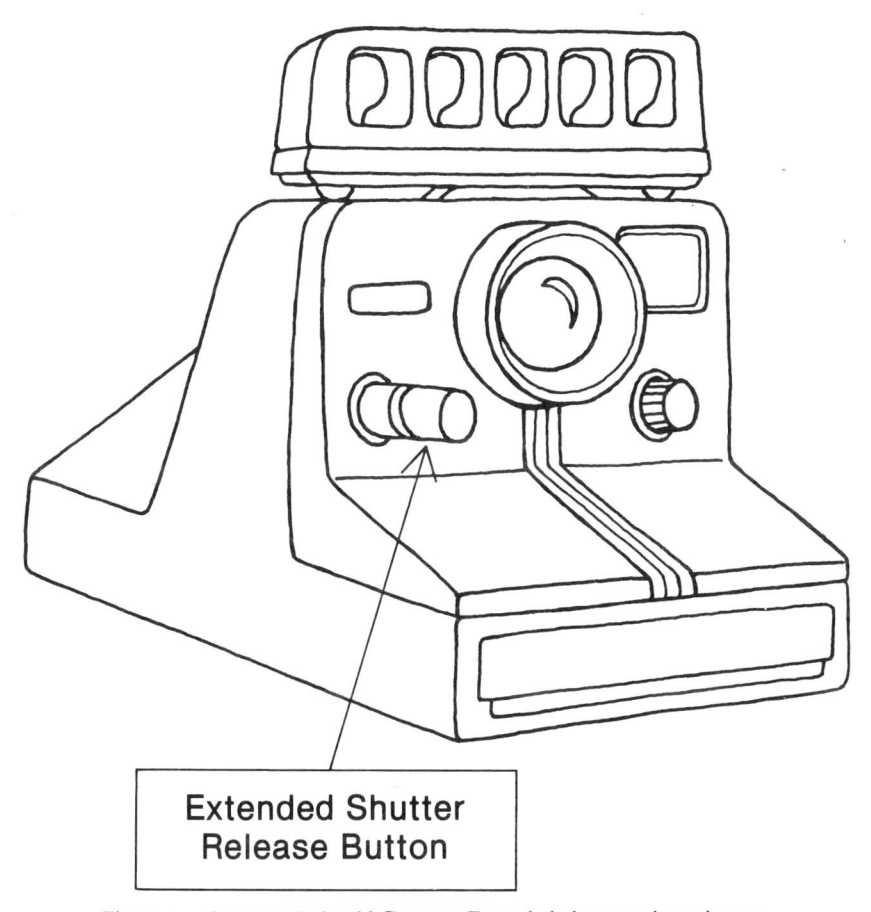

Figure 1. One-step Polaroid Camera: Extended shutter release button.

environments: outdoors in a residential neighborhood three city blocks from the agency; in a community park; in the Virginia Museum; and in the participant's home. The participant was informed, prior to leaving the developmental center for the probe, that she would be required to take photographs at the location.

Instructional Design

The photography study incorporated a test-teach design (Brown, 1973) with daily data collection. This design included an initial baseline to determine preinstruction competence. This was followed by a period of instruction. After criterion performance was reached, generalization probes were taken across four other environments.

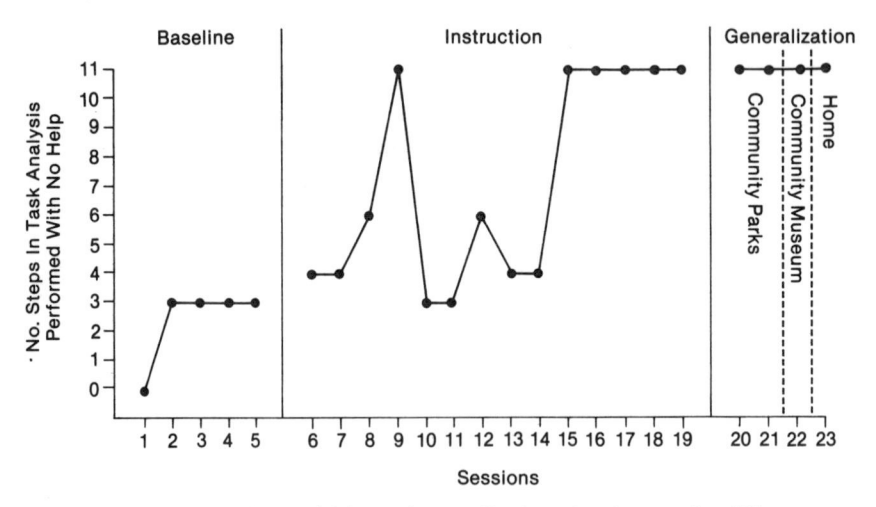

Figure 2. Ruth: acquisition and generalization of a photography skill.

Results

Inspection of Ruth's responses shows a relatively stable baseline. She did not perform any of the steps successfully on the first day and performed three steps of the skill without assistance during the baseline's remainder. Figure 2 illustrates the number of steps of the task analysis performed independently during baseline, instruction, and generalization probes.

The graph displays that once instruction was initated, the participant immediately improved performance. After 11 training sessions, criterion for mastery of the photography skill was attained. As can be seen, all steps were performed independently during session nine, but similar performance was not exhibited during the subsequent session. Therefore, training continued until Ruth mastered all 11 steps for five consecutive sessions (15–19).

As can be seen on Figure 2, sessions 20-23, she was able to complete all the steps required and successfully took two photographs at each location. These trials were intrinsically rewarding, as upon arrival to the agency each time, Ruth was unusually verbal and proudly displayed the photographs to all staff and several other clients.

Discussion

The results of this brief case study provide a model for effectively integrating programmatic adaptations with systematic instruction principles. It also describes the addition of a leisure skill that is chronologically age appropriate; previous skills had involved ball play and inappropriate table activities. The staff in the center and parents began to see Ruth as a more competent individual, since nonhandicapped persons also enjoy picture taking activity.

CASE STUDY II: DEVELOPING INDEPENDENT COOKING SKILLS IN A PROFOUNDLY RETARDED WOMAN

One skill area that has received limited attention and yet is critical to independence or semi-independence in group homes, supervised apartments, or real homes is cooking and meal preparation. A review of literature indicated that only a study by Robinson-Wilson (1976) addressed this important area. The focus of this program was the use of picture recipes as a means of facilitating meal preparation skills.

Cooking as an instructional goal may have a threefold objective. First, it may be a necessary skill to acquire for eating independently. Second, it can be an excellent leisure activity, for once an individual acquires general stove-use skills, many types of foods and meals may be prepared. Third, cooking skills are frequently required in many hotel and restaurant settings for kitchen job vacancies.

The purpose of this program was to train a profoundly mentally retarded woman in three specific cooking skills, with a focus on these skills being used for leisure activity. Systematic instructional procedures were used in combination with a series of material and procedural modifications.

Participant

Heidi is a 28 year old adult female attending an adult development center. Her IQ on the Stanford-Binet is 19, placing her in the profoundly retarded range. According to her AAMD classification, her adaptive functioning is in the severely retarded range. Heidi is an epileptic, having daily petit and grand mal seizures. She receives the following medications and dosages for the control of her seizures: mysoline, 250 mg, three times daily; tegretol, 200 mg, three times daily; and dilantin, 300 mg, once daily.

Heidi's frequent loud and inappropriate verbalizations are disruptive to others in the immediate environment. Her receptive language is good. Her expressive language, however, is poor: she exhibits high degrees of perseveratory speech. Heidi is inconsistent in her performance on most tasks. High distractability negatively affects most efforts at instruction and performance is facilitated only in a one-to-one trainer/staff situation. Heidi responds well to social reinforcement (e.g., verbal praise, hugs, back rubs) although she rarely initiates any activity.

Following conversation with parents and observation in the participant's home, it was discovered that Heidi's free time consisted of completing simple chores in the home (e.g., getting ashtrays for guests), singing childrens' songs while dancing inappropriately by herself, and watching her mother prepare meals.

Setting

Instruction took place at a community adult development center in the greater Richmond, Virginia area. The center offers daily living, social/communication, and vocational skills training to 12 severely and profoundly handicapped persons over 21 years of age. The clients attend the center daily from 9 a.m. to 3 p.m. The cooking program transpired in the center's kitchen area. This room contained cooking materials and appliances commonly found in the home environment (e.g., stove, sink, counter top, refrigerator/freezer, coffeemaker, cupboards, cooking utensils).

Program Objective

The objective of this program was to develop and evaluate cooking skills in a severely retarded adult. Three skills were targeted for instruction, each utilizing a different function of a kitchen stove. Boiling an egg requires manipulation of the top stove burner, broiling an English muffin and cheese utilizes the oven broiler, and a TV dinner requires use of the baking oven. To reach criterion on each skill, the participant had to perform each step of a task analysis correctly and without assistance on two consecutive days. Upon completion of the cooking program, Heidi would be able to prepare three meals successfully and independently.

Secondary objectives were to generalize the cooking skills to two other environments (i.e., another community training facility that Heidi would be transferring to in the near future, participant's home) and to the preparation of other recipes requiring similar skills and behaviors (i.e., boil frozen vegetable cooking bag, broil hot dog, bake frozen pizza). The generalization of skills to the preparation of additional dishes would make the program cost effective. With a simple verbal prompt including an action verb (e.g., "Heidi, broil the hot dog."), the participant could prepare several dishes with mastery of just a few skills.

Rationale for Skill Selection

The rationale for selection of the three cooking skills was that a) Heidi previously enjoyed observing her mother prepare the family dinners and snacks; b) by teaching skills employing three distinct uses of a kitchen stove, potential for the preparation of a wider variety of meals is made possible (for example, instead of teaching cooking skills using the top stove burner exclusively, and limiting the individual's repertoire to the generalization of other boiling recipes, cooking skills from each of the three oven modes may allow for a more versatile cook and potential for much greater generalization); c) the equipment was available in the training center and home; d) cooking activities are functional, chronologically age appropriate, and are daily living skills that facilitate independent community living.

Materials and Equipment/Special Adaptations

The materials employed in the program are commensurate with those commonly used in a domestic kitchen. Special adaptations were implemented when necessary to simplify the cooking skills using readily available household items. Cost, safety, and convenience were considered when designing the program. Hard boiled eggs were used during the boiling skill, eliminating breakage and allowing for repeated use of one egg. An empty TV dinner tray covered with aluminum foil was placed in its original carton and used in place of a real dinner. This eliminated the spillage of boiling liquids and sauces from the tray and was cost effective.

Additional modified materials/equipment included a color coded stove with a separate heat control knob that could be simply manipulated by the instructor, and a portable kitchen timer with a removable red tape strip for correct cooking time identification. Other materials/equipment and special adaptations are listed in Table 2.

Experimental Design

The program incorporated a multiple baseline design across the three different cooking skills. Preinstruction competencies were determined by initial baselines. Baseline data were collected across each skill after which instruction commenced on boiling an egg. During the instruction phase of this skill, baselining continued on the English muffin and TV dinner skills. A minimal competency level of a five-step increase on the task analysis for two consecutive trials led to instruction on the following skill. Baseline continued on the final skill until the same minimal competency level was obtained on broiling the English muffin and cheese. At this time, instruction began on baking the TV dinner. Criterion for mastery of a skill was 100 percent independent performance of all the steps of the task analysis on two consecutive trials. Following acquisition of Skills A and B, weekly probes were taken until criterion was met on Skill C.

Procedure

Instruction was conducted four to five times per week, with approximately 15 minutes of instruction per skill. Sessions were held in the late morning hours prior to lunch because the cooking skills could be appropriate as lunchtime meal preparation.

A different task analysis was utilized to identify component subskills of each cooking activity. Table 3 includes the task analysis, performance

Table 2. Materials and special adaptations for three cooking skills

Skill	Materials/Equipment	Modification
Boil egg	Egg	Hard-boiled egg (prevent breakage)
	Saucepan full of boiling water	Place egg into empty saucepan, then fill with water
	Water	—
	Stove: top stove burner	Color-coded dial and burner; cover extraneous dials with placemats (to facilitate match-to-sample)
	Kitchen timer	Red tape strip (mark appropriate calibrations)
	Spoon	Slotted spoon (prevent scalding, easier to recover egg)
	Bowl	Extra large plastic salad bowl (prevent breakage, increase chance for accuracy)
Broil English muffin and cheese	English muffin	—
	Cheese slice	Presliced American cheese
	Aluminum foil	Pie pan to simplify manipulation of muffin
	Stove: broiler	Color-coded dial and broiler door; cover extraneous dials with placemats
	Kitchen timer	Red tape strip
	Pot holder	Glove pot holder (ensure safety)
Bake TV dinner	TV dinner	Empty TV dinner tray covered with aluminum foil (economically feasible)
	Stove: oven	Color-coded dial and oven door; cover extraneous dials with placemats
	Kitchen timer	Red tape strip
	Pot holder	Glove pot holder

Table 3. Task analyses for three cooking skills

I. Boiling Egg
   Performance Objective: Given the appropriate cooking materials and kitchen stove (top burner), the participant will boil the egg until hard boiled with 100% proficiency on 2 consecutive days.
   Verbal Cue: "Heidi, boil the egg."
   1. Place egg in saucepan without breaking it.
   2. Lift saucepan off stove with nondominant hand using palmar grasp, and position directly under water faucet.
   3. Turn water on with dominant hand to fill saucepan 1/2 full and turn off water.
   4. Place saucepan onto top stove burner.
   5. Turn on burner underneath saucepan.
   6. Set electric timer for 15 minutes.
   7. Wait for timer to ring.
   8. Turn off burner.

Table 3. (*Continued*)

    9. Remove egg from saucepan using slotted spoon.
   10. Place egg in bowl.
II. Broiling English Muffin and Cheese
    Performance Objective: Given the appropriate cooking materials and kitchen stove (broiler), the participant will broil the English muffin and cheese with 100% proficiency on 2 consecutive days.
    Verbal Cue: "Heidi, broil the English muffin and cheese."
    1. Place slice of cheese on English muffin half.
    2. Place prepared muffin onto oven tray.
    3. Open broiler door.
    4. Place tray on top rack in oven.
    5. Close broiler door three-quarters way to first stop position.
    6. Turn oven knob all the way to "broil."
    7. Set electric timer for 5 minutes.
    8. Wait for timer to ring.
    9. Turn off broiler.
   10. Place pot holder glove on each hand.
   11. Open broiler door.
   12. Pull oven rack out halfway exposing oven tray.
   13. Remove tray from broiler (with palm facing upward) and place on stove top.
   14. Close broiler door.
III. Baking TV Dinner
    Performance Objective: Given the appropriate cooking materials and kitchen stove (oven), the participant will bake the TV dinner with 100% proficiency on 2 consecutive days.
    Verbal Cue: "Heidi, bake the TV dinner."
    1. Remove dinner from carton.
    2. Open oven door using nondominant hand and place TV dinner on bottom rack.
    3. Close oven door all the way.
    4. Turn oven temperature knob to 425°.
    5. Set electric timer for 40 minutes.
    6. Wait for timer to ring (participant should leave kitchen and resume other activity during this time).
    7. When timer rings, turn oven temperature knob to "off" position.
    8. Place pot holder glove on each hand.
    9. Open oven door.
   10. Pull oven rack out halfway exposing TV dinner.
   12. Close oven door.

objective, and verbal cue for each skill. A popular cook book, *Joy of Cooking* (Rombauer & Rombauer-Becker, 1964) and center staff consultation assisted in the development of the task analyses. It was evident following staff discussions concerning the capabilities of the participant, that various procedural modifications were necessary if the skills were to be successfully acquired by Heidi. For example, the task analysis for boiling an egg initially required the egg to be placed in a saucepan and then the pan to be filled with water. This was preferred to the alternate method of placing the egg into boiling water. The former method was safer and also reduced egg breakage. Incorporated into the boiling and baking task analyses for safety reasons was the manipulation of the oven rack and employment of an underhand method to remove the food items to avoid arm contact with the heating coils located at the top of the oven.

The baseline performance levels for each skill were determined by giving the general verbal cue (e.g., "Heidi, boil the egg.") and recording the number of steps performed independently. One baseline trial was conducted per session for each skill.

Following initial baseline, the trainer began instruction on the next step of the task analysis on boiling egg, which had not been performed correctly on two consecutive trials. Instruction utilized a three step cue hierarchy ranging from least to most intrusive. This instructional strategy was found to be an effective teaching method in a previous leisure skills program with a severely handicapped adult (Wehman, Schleien, & Kiernan, Note 1). The trainer provided the verbal cue and socially reinforced an appropriate response. If an incorrect response occurred, the second step of the cue hierarchy was implemented. At this time, the verbal cue was repeated while the trainer modeled the correct behavior. Social reinforcement was provided for a correct response. Failure to elicit the desired response led to the final step of the hierarchy, which entailed the trainer once again giving the verbal cue and physically guiding the participant through the correct behavior, after which praise was given.

Five training trials on the targeted step were performed each session. Following instruction, the general verbal cue was given and the participant's behaviors recorded. No modeling or physical prompting was offered during the nonreinforced probes. Weekly probes were conducted following mastery of the skills to ensure endurance of performance until all skills were mastered and generalized.

A reliability check was taken by a second recorder twice per week. Interobserver reliability averaged 0.97 across the three cooking skills.

Results and Discussion

The participant learned to prepare all three meals in the cooking program following a multiple baseline design. Figure 3 illustrates the number of the task analyses performed correctly during baseline, instruction, weekly probes, and generalization for each cooking skill. Daily stable baseline rates were obtained for each skill, clearly demonstrating Heidi's low competency levels (e.g., 0-step proficiency during boiling an egg baseline) in this leisure area.

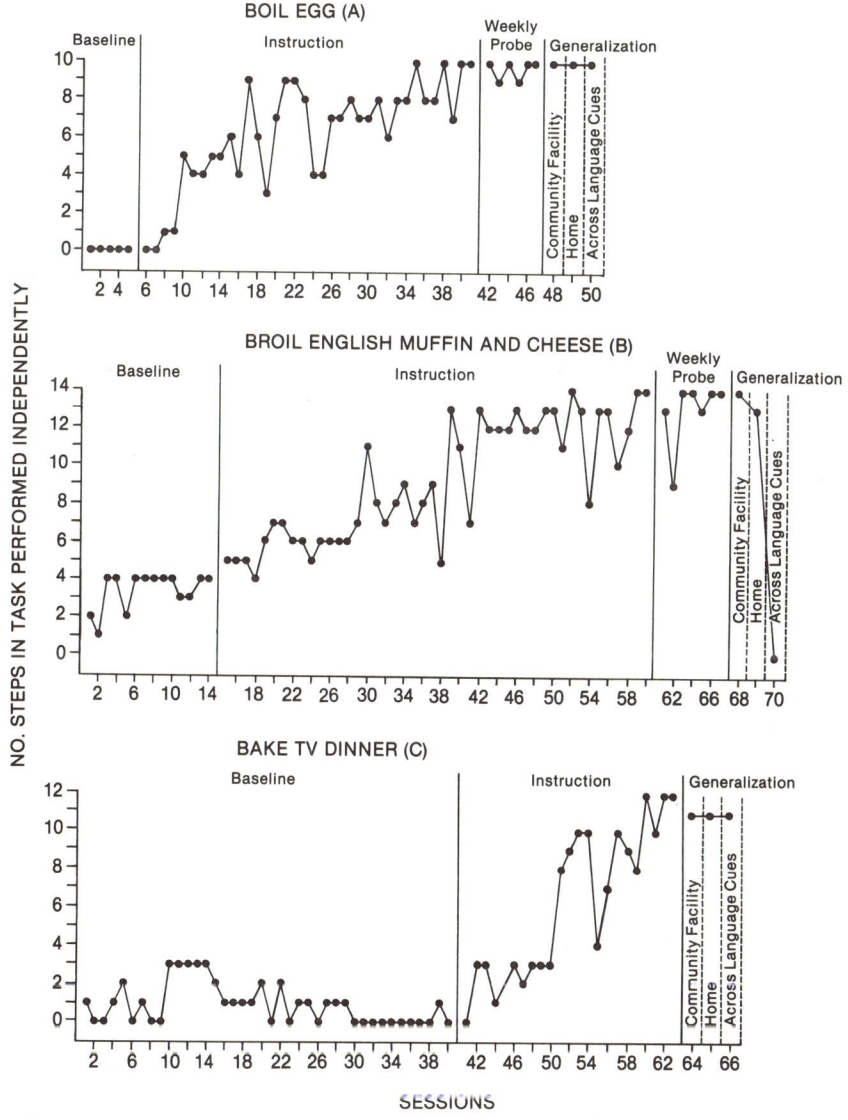

Figure 3. Number of steps in three cooking skills performed independently by Heidi.

Boiling an egg, broiling an English muffin and cheese, and baking a TV dinner were instructed in that order. This skill sequence was chosen by staff because of its increasing level of difficulty. Although there was a general increase in the number of steps performed independently throughout instruction, a jagged profile appears due to the participant's frequent seizures. Seizures occurring during instruction impaired performance significantly. However, Heidi frequently upgraded her performance on the following day and occasionally exceeded her previous competency level. This resulted in the eventual acquisition of the skills. Number of sessions for skill acquisition varied from 23 to 46.

Weekly probes demonstrated the endurance of the participant's cooking performance while training was still in progress on the other skills. The results of the generalization probes were twofold: they demonstrated Heidi's ability to cook in other environments (i.e., another community training center, participant's home) using different cooking facilities, and second, the participant acquired the skills necessary for two general uses of an oven (i.e., boiling, baking), as well as three specific skills of boiling an egg, broiling a muffin, and baking a TV dinner.

The results of the present study clearly demonstrate the functional relationship between the systematic instructional procedures and materials/skill modification and the acquisition of different cooking skills. Since baselines on the second and third skills remained at low rates until intervention occurred, it is evident that the instructional program led to the development of these cooking skills in Heidi.

Generalization probes suggest that Heidi was able to transfer use of a stove, both to other environments (i.e., another community facility, participant's home) and across language cues (i.e., boil cooking packet, bake pizza). An attempt to generalize the broiling skill using a hot dog achieved negative results. This could have been due to a poor selection of food items, since Heidi had previously been exposed to the boiling of hot dogs in the home. It may have been Heidi's logical assumption that the hot dogs be prepared in boiling water and not in the broiler. Eleven of the 12 steps were performed independently across the three generalization probes for baking and she successfully performed 13 of the 14 steps on the broiling skill in the home. It is believed that although performance on these trials did not reach 100%, it did represent a significant increase over preinstruction ability. Furthermore, as was demonstrated when Heidi baked a pizza, a sufficient number of steps of the task analysis were performed correctly in order for her to independently cook a complete snack.

CASE STUDY III: GROUP HOME LEISURE PROGRAMMING

Our third case study is directed toward group home leisure programming for handicapped adults. If group homes are to be a successful aspect of residential services, then leisure education will play a major role. Instruction and guidance in this area is necessary to promote independence and avoid inappropriate antisocial behavior that will reduce acceptance by nonhandicapped neighbors. One aspect of optimal personal and social adjustments for retarded individuals is the capacity to use free time appropriately, constructively, or creatively. Therefore, a leisure program was designed for a local group home serving mentally retarded adults in Richmond, Virginia. The purposes of this study were threefold: a) to develop and implement a program that had instructional elements that were easily replicable by other group home staff; b) to develop a program that evaluated *quality* of resident leisure behaviors; and c) to evaluate the program in an experimental design that allowed for the verification of the instructional package employed.

Participants and Setting

Six residents of a community group home for mentally retarded adults participated in the leisure program. The participants, each classified as moderately mentally retarded, were three males and three females ranging from 27 to 52 years of age. The majority were from institutional backgrounds and exhibited inappropriate stereotypic social behaviors (e.g., nonfunctional perseverations, inappropriate conversation/silly talk, aimless wandering, difficulty establishing and maintaining social relationships). Two residents lived at home with their families in socially impoverished environments prior to the group home placement and were similarly deficient in appropriate social behavior and leisure skills.

Behavior Observations

Systematic observations of the participants' behaviors during their leisure or free time were made to serve as preintervention baseline. In this manner, accurate and objective assessments were made of the participants' leisure skill repertoires. Data were taken over 5 consecutive weeknights between 7:30 and 8:30 p.m. This interval, which followed dinner and cleanup, was agreed upon by group home staff and participants as the most appropriate and feasible time for programming leisure skills. This time period was held constant throughout all phases of the program.

Observers/Counselors and Reliability

Nine rotating observers were employed in the program. Five were Virginia Commonwealth University, Department of Special Education undergraduate students, two were group home staff, and the remainder were master's degree level project staff. Two trained observers were present at the home each night and stationed at high frequency recreation areas (i.e., living room, basement TV/game room). The observers were introduced as friends of the group home staff, as this would not significantly alter the residents' leisure time behaviors. Clipboards were not used and observational data forms were placed inside magazines and kept out of sight. When queried by participants as to the purpose of their presence, they replied they were doing homework. The two project staff members led the leisure counseling sessions.

A reliability check was made by a third trained observer one night per week. Interobserver reliability ranged from 70 to 100% with a mean of 0.87. Each observer was responsible for recording behaviors of three participants. The third observer made recordings concurrently with one of the regular observers on the same three participants and data were compared. The night of the week and observer checked were arbitrarily selected.

A momentary time sampling technique was employed in order to record quality of leisure behavior of the six residents. At 15 second intervals, the behavior that the participant was eliciting at that moment was recorded. Each participant was observed consecutively. Thus, a total of 80 recordings were made on every participant per evening. Following a week of baseline, each participant had been observed for 400 intervals.

Three categories of behaviors were operationally defined and coded for the assessment process. The three classifications, high quality (HQ) and low quality (LQ) leisure behavior, and inappropriate (I) social behavior are defined in Table 4. These behavioral categories were determined by group home staff following a prebaseline observation period. During this time, all behaviors elicited by the participants were listed, and staff discussion concerning their quality followed. Representative behaviors falling under each of the three classifications are also provided in Table 4.

Experimental Design

An ABAB reversal design was employed. This was composed of the following four phases: phase I (baseline); phase II (instruction/reinforcement); phase III (return to baseline, in which instruction and reinforcement were withheld); and phase IV (instruction/reinforcement reinstated). Each phase is described in detail below.

Phase I (Baseline) Behavioral observations were made in the group home in order to determine preinstruction leisure skill behavior patterns and competencies. This phase consisted of 5 days. Observers used the table of operational definitions and examples of leisure behaviors to determine the classification of the elicited behaviors.

Phase II (Instruction/Reinforcement) Exposure to new and chronologically age appropriate, leisure related materials and equipment began simultaneously with leisure counseling instruction. Materials and equipment introduced included: playing cards, dart set, jigsaw puzzles, Carrom Billiards set, silk screening materials, computerized "Odyssey" TV game, and a guitar.

Table 4. Operational definitions of leisure behaviors

High Quality Leisure Behavior (HQ)
*Goal-directed recreational activity (includes goal-directed conversation relevant to leisure).
*Chronologically age-appropriate.
*Appropriate use of materials and/or equipment in a manner consistent with current level of training.
(*note: All criteria listed above must be met in order for behavior to be considered high quality.)

Representative behaviors:[a] Speaking on telephone, looking through book/magazine, taking photographs with camera, use of photo album, playing cards, assembling jigsaw puzzle, dancing with partner, watering plants, cooking/preparing snack.

Low Quality Leisure Behavior (LQ)
Use of leisure related materials and/or equipment in a manner inconsistent with present level of training.
Sitting or lying passively without participating in an activity.
Watching television.
Smoking without additional activity.
Solitary engagement in an appropriate activity that necessarily requires more than one participant.

Representative behaviors:[a] Television on and not watching, holding book/magazine without perusal, dancing alone, strumming guitar without making chords, staring out window, sitting and doing nothing.

Inappropriate Social Behavior (I)
Inappropriate use of materials.
Use of chronologically age-inappropriate materials (determined by manufacturer's recommended age level).
Violently aggressive verbal or physical behavior.
Nongoal-directed, nonfunctional, purposeless behavior (e.g., wandering aimlessly around home, spinning in circles).
Purposeless, nonsensical conversation (e.g., speaking to oneself, speaking to another individual in a socially unacceptable manner, echolalic or perseverative speech).
Stereotypic behavior (e.g., body rocking, self-stimulation).
Behavior out of context.

Representative behaviors:[a] Manipulating child's popcorn popper toy, talking to self, listening to dial tone on telephone, throwing deck of cards across room, bowling with miniature toy set, walking across room with book balanced on head, continuous pacing across room.

[a] If observed behavior is not listed as representative behavior, it must meet above criteria to be considered in its respective category.

Instruction consisted of a weekly leisure education group counseling session. These sessions were 1 hour in length, except for an initial session of 2 hours. Leisure counseling was designed as a preparation for community leisure pursuits. A hierarchy was utilized to attain this goal. The first of six sessions was a directed discussion of recreational pursuits and past and present leisure/free time use. The counselor initiated group conversation concerning many philosophical aspects of recreation (i.e., past recreational experiences, present leisure repertoires, activity preferences, and generally, the purpose for and benefits of recreational participation). Additionally, categories of recreation (e.g., games, hobbies, sports) were compared and contrasted and their individual relevancies discussed, for example, a daily jogging program as a hobby and a viable means for the release of pent-up energies.

The second hierarchical step of the counseling program lasted three sessions and entailed general skill instruction relevant to the newly introduced materials. Residents were encouraged to participate and practice during their own time throughout each week to enhance skill acquisition. Playing rules were taught within the context of the activities. The card games "Concentration" and "I Doubt It" were learned by participating with the counselors, instructors, and peers. Modeling was used to teach skills and appropriate social interactions during participation.

The final phase of the counseling hierarchy involved the preparation of the participants for actual engagement in activity within the community. This strategy is consistent with the group homes' ultimate goal of normalized and independent community recreational involvement. To achieve this goal, individuals had to acquire specific skills necessary for participation in community-based activities. An adult must have the ability to select an activity independently and self-initiate performance, as well as interact and cooperate with fellow participants. In order to self-initiate, one must pursue activities commensurate with his or her strengths and weaknesses. This requires not only familiarity with the activity in question but a sense of the individual's abilities and talents. Beyond the playing rules necessary for specific activity, there are guidelines that must be adhered to when recreating with peers, especially when in the community. These social interaction factors must also be considered when preparing the individual for normalized participation outside the home agency.

To incorporate these necessary components of community participation, an instructional program was developed using tournament play. During the fifth instructional session, the counselors announced that a leisure skills tournament was to begin in the group home. The activities on the tournament program included darts (adapted "Cricket"), "Carrom Billiards," playing cards ("Concentration," "I Doubt It," "Baseball"), and art (modeling clay, silk screening, jigsaw puzzles). These activities were jointly decided upon by the counselors, participants, and group home staff.

Homemade scoreboards were used and appropriate activity stations designated. Participants were encouraged to keep score for themselves in the various skills or to ask staff for assistance in recording points when necessary. Points were assigned to activities on the basis of time and effort expended. In this manner, participation would be based on the individual's interests and preferences, as opposed to a quick point payoff. Participants were informed that awards would be given for competency in the various activity areas. The awards (i.e., award pins, certificates) were put on display at the commencement of tournament play. The tournament lasted 3 weeks at the end of which an awards presentation was held. At this time, participants received their awards in the presence of peers and staff.

Reinforcement Schedule As well as the weekly counseling periods, data collection/reinforcement sessions were implemented. These occurred 3 nights per week and entailed use of a variable interval schedule. Each session lasted 1 hour and was divided into 10 data collection/reinforcement intervals, resulting in a variable interval schedule averaging one reinforcement every 6 minutes (see Table 5).

If a participant was engaging in high quality leisure behavior (HQ) at one of these predetermined intervals, he or she would be socially

Table 5. Variable interval reinforcement schedule (VI-6[a])

Program begins	7:30 p.m.	
	7:33 p.m.	R+[b]
	7:37 p.m.	R+
	7:43 p.m.	R+
Nonreinforced probe	7:45–7:55 p.m.	
	7:56 p.m.	R+
	8:05 p.m.	R+
	8:08 p.m.	R+
	8:12 p.m.	R+
Nonreinforced probe	8:14–8:24 p.m.	
	8:25 p.m.	R+
	8:27 p.m.	R+
	8:29 p.m.	R+

[a] (VI-6): On the average, each 6 minutes, participant gets reinforced for high quality (HQ) leisure behavior.

[b] R+ denotes: positive social reinforcement.

reinforced by the instructor. Reinforcement consisted of praise, encouragement, and actual participation by the instructor alongside the participant for a period of 1 minute. If the individual was engaging in low quality leisure (LQ) or inappropriate (I) behavior at one of the data points, reinforcement was withheld. Leisure performance was observed and recorded at each of the 10 intervals, resulting in 10 data points per session.

During seven of the data collection/reinforcement sessions, nonreinforced behavior probes were taken. These consisted of two 10 minute observation periods per session. Within each period, each participant was observed consecutively at 15 second intervals. Behavior (i.e., HQ, LQ, I) was then recorded but no reinforcement was administered.

Phase III (Return to Baseline Following 17 instructional sessions, a return to baseline was implemented. This entailed 1 week (3 sessions) without counseling or any reinforcement for high quality leisure behavior. Materials and equipment were available during this time. Data collection was carried out in the same manner as during the instructional sessions using nonreinforced probes for all three sessions. Data collectors unfamiliar to the participants took data during this phase. This eliminated incidental reinforcing elements associated with the regular data collectors.

Phase IV (Instruction/Reinforcement Reinstated) During the final phase of the program, instruction and reinforcement were reinstated. One counseling and five data collection/reinforcement sessions were held. Nonreinforced probes were also made during the hourly data collection periods.

Results and Discussion

It is evident from the initial baseline observations in Figure 4 that there was minimal high quality leisure behavior (HQ) present among the six group home residents. The most prevalent leisure activities engaged in during that time included watching television and smoking cigarettes. Included among the preinstructional recreational materials present in the home were a child's popcorn popper toy, miniature plastic bowling set, unopened pack of playing cards, television, radio, and a broken and inoperable table tennis set.

Following the initial counseling session and exposure to only one new material (i.e., dart set), the mean percentage of HQ significantly increased from a baseline mean of 5.6% to 40%. At no time during instruction did the mean percentage of HQ fall below the 40% mark. HQ averaged 60% across the 17 instruction/reinforcement sessions. During instruction, on the average, both LQ and I decreased significantly.

When HQ reached its peak percentage at 94%, a return to baseline was instituted. At this time HQ immediately dropped significantly and continued to steadily decline.

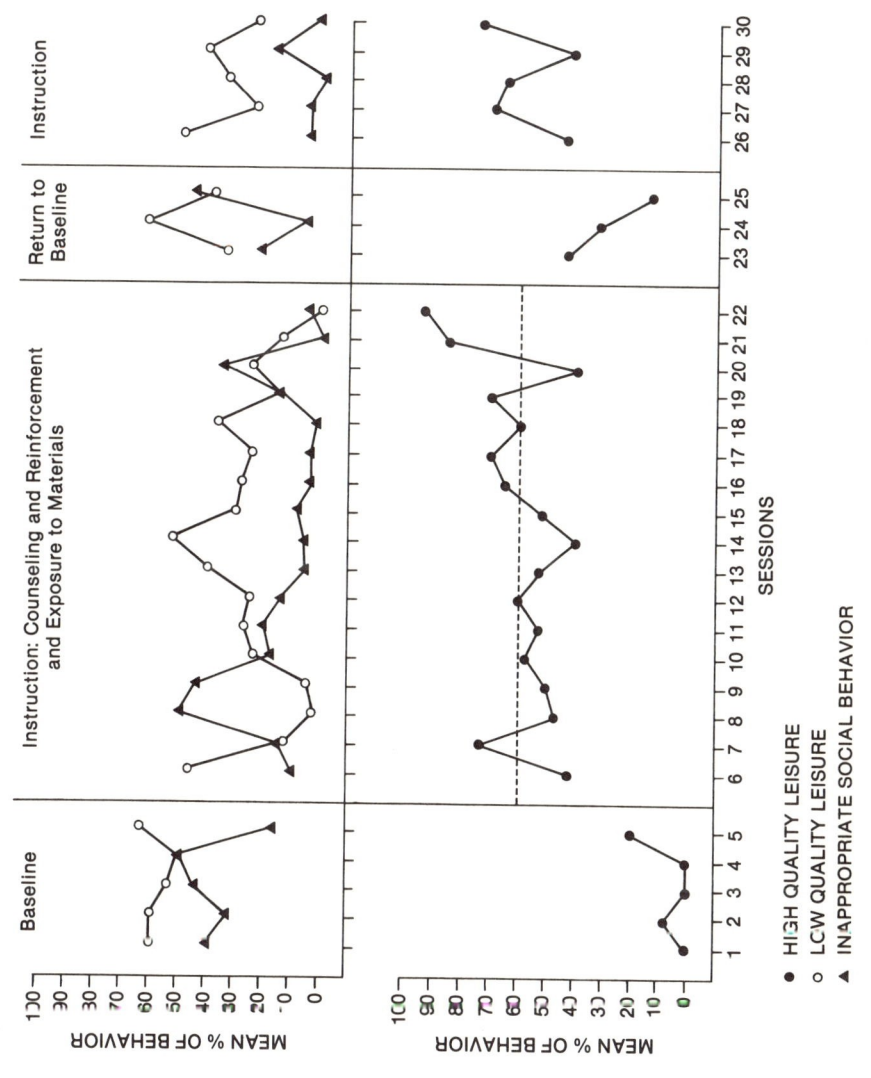

Figure 4. Mean percentage of leisure behavior of group home participants.

After instruction was reinstated, HQ once again rose to the original instruction phase level. Inappropriate behavior decreased to a level approaching 0%. It is quite evident that throughout the leisure programming period, there was an inverse relationship between HQ and I. Individuals recreating appropriately had little time for antisocial, stereotypic, or age-inappropriate behavior. This is in support of Favell's (1973) research concerning the reduction of stereotypes through the acquisition of leisure skills.

The present study demonstrated several positive points. First, a traditionally underserved population of moderately mentally retarded adults participated in a leisure program that provided chronologically age-appropriate objects and activities. Second, the intervention "package" of counseling, social reinforcement, and availability of materials was identified as an effective means of facilitating leisure skills. Third, the intervention program was shown to have a functional relationship with high quality activity; concurrently, inappropriate social behaviors were reduced in most of the residents.

A primary implication to be drawn from this program is that group home residents need not engage only in passive and low-quality leisure activities. This study presents a model that community residential staff can utilize in their respective programs. The components for instructional intervention have been delineated clearly for replication; the time of a professional therapeutic recreation specialist should be required only weekly.

CASE STUDY IV: TEACHING MULTIHANDICAPPED ADULTS DART SKILLS

In this last case study, we have demonstrated the development of dart throwing skills in severely and profoundly retarded adults. This chronologically age appropriate program was undertaken to help the participants learn leisure skills that could be used in the community. The program was evaluated in a combination changing criteria and multiple baseline design.

Setting and Participants

The participants were three multihandicapped individuals attending a community adult development center. The agency offers self-help, social/communication, and prevocational skills training to 12 severely and profoundly handicapped persons between 21 and 63 years of age. The clients attend the center from 9 a.m. to 3 p.m. Monday through Friday. The darts skills leisure training program transpired in the recreation room within the complex. The three participants, each with varying degrees of physical and intellectual deficits, are described below.

Participant 1: Herman is a 63 year old black male. He has cerebral palsy (athetoid type) an unsteady, uncoordinated gait with poor dynamic and static balance. The participant has difficulty visually tracking moving objects. Arm/leg extension and flexion are additionally poor. Herman has an IQ of 27 on the Stanford-Binet placing him in the severely retarded range. His AAMD Adaptive Behavior Scale scores are also at the severe level. His verbal communication skills are inadequate. Expressive language is limited, although his receptive language skills allow him to follow multiple step directions. The participant's vocational skills potential is inadequate for a sheltered workshop placement. Since his parents are deceased, Herman lives with his niece and her husband. His guardians and development center staff report that Herman's level of functioning has deteriorated in recent years. The participant once enjoyed perusing illustrated magazines, taking neighborhood walks, and engaging in simple card games. However, these skills and interests have ceased, and his present leisure skills repertoire consists of merely smoking approximately three packs of cigarettes daily and watching television in the evening hours.

Participant 2: Roselyn is a 32 year old white female. She is cerebral palsied (spastic type) with severely contracted muscles in her right arm giving her no fine and minimal gross motor movements. Coordination in her left arm is somewhat better with a modified pincer grasp. Due to a dislocated right hip, Roselyn is unable to stand unsupported and requires a walker for locomotion. Additionally, her arm/leg extension and flexion are limited on her right side. She has an IQ of 35 on the Stanford-Binet placing her in the moderately retarded range. Her social functioning on the AAMD Adaptive Behavior Scale is high relative to her other areas of functioning. Roselyn's expressive language skills are poor to moderate. Her behavioral affect is lethargic. Motivation level is low and she seldom initiates activity. Due to her retarded motoric functioning resulting in low production rates, a sheltered workshop has not been an appropriate placement to date. During her unobligated time, Roselyn enjoys attending professional hockey games and movies, but these community facilities are accessible only when her parents or relatives are willing to accompany and transport her. Although she enjoys spectator/passive recreational activity, Roselyn lacks specific skills necessary to participate in active and age-appropriate leisure skills.

Participant 3: Robert is a 23 year old white male. He is Down's Syndrome profoundly retarded. The participant obtained a Stanford-Binet IQ score of 8 and is categorized as nontrainable. Center staff have reported that Robert has yet to maintain, generalize, or initiate any behavior that he has acquired within 2 years of attendance at the agency. His behavioral functioning is described as autistic, demonstrating perseverative, self-stimulatory motor movements and other stereotypic behavior (e.g., body rocking, placing hands in front of face, staring aimlessly). Speech consists exclusively of delayed echolalia and spontaneous verbal behavior is nonexistent. Robert is visually impaired, requiring special eyeglass lenses. He is a diabetic and requires daily doses of insulin and restricted diet. The participant is unable to follow one-step directions and lacks the cognitive skills of object permanence and the realization of means/end. He is often noncompliant, requiring continuous physical prompting to complete most tasks. Robert is occasionally physically aggressive and has been known to strike his peers. Moderate success in eliciting operant responses has been found through the use of social and edible reinforcement. Robert does not engage in any leisure related activity.

Program Objective

The objective of the dart skills leisure program was for each participant to throw three darts and successfully strike the dartboard each toss from the standard 8-foot distance. Criteria for mastery consisted of 100% completion of the seven step task analysis for two consecutive sessions.

An additional objective of the program was to generalize dart throwing performance to three other environments (i.e., community dart bar, staff's apartment, another training facility). The goal of the generalization probes was to elicit criterion level performance in the other, more normal, environments using just a verbal prompt. During these nonreinforced probes, if the participant did not perform at an acceptable level (i.e., two of three darts striking board), instruction would be reinstated in the generalized environment.

Skill Selection Validity

The rationale for selection of the dart game was fourfold: 1) *age appropriateness*—standard dart games are considered by the community to be chronologically age-appropriate; 2) *competing behaviors*—recreation staff strongly desired to eliminate play with a child's dart set using velcro balls by one of the adults by instructing and substituting a more appropriate and acceptable behavior; 3) *social validity*—it was noted via informal survey that 25% of the bars in the local community contain a minimum of one dartboard (apparently a popular pastime in the Richmond area); and 4) *therapeutic*—since two of the participants are physically handicapped (i.e., cerebral palsy), dart tossing facilitates eye-hand coordination and potential for number recognition skills. Additionally, the third participant is provided a means for physical expression to compensate for

Table 6. Participants' existing motor skills versus basic skills necessary for dart toss

Participants' skills			Minimum motor skills: Darts
Herman	Roselyn	Robert	
×	×	×	1. Head erect
×		×	2. Stand/sit unsupported
×	×[a]	×	3. Pincer grasp (one hand)
×	×	×	4. Arm flexion (one arm)
×	×	×	5. Arm extension (one arm)
×	×	×	6. Controlled hand release (one hand)
×	×		7. Visual tracking
×[b]	×[b]	×	8. Eye-hand coordination

[a] Modified pincer grasp.
[b] Limited eye-hand coordination due to cerebral palsy.

a lack of verbal expression. Table 6 contrasts the existing motor skills of the participants to the basic core skills that facilitate participation in this particular leisure activity (i.e., dart toss).

Procedure

Instruction was 15 minutes per participant daily and was conducted five times per week. Sessions were held at different times throughout each day in order for the participant to easily generalize the skills to any time of day. Additionally, this training regime allowed the clients to utilize this recreational activity during their break time from development center prevocational training.

A seven step task analysis was used for instruction. Content validity was established through observations of competitors in a tournament throwing darts in a community darts bar by a therapeutic recreation specialist. Besides the basic motor skills required to grasp, aim, and toss a dart (e.g., pincer grasp, arm flexion/extension, controlled hand release), 100% accuracy in striking the dartboard was required for mastery of the skill. The rationale for this seemingly stringent minimal criterion level was twofold. First of all, most dart players usually strike the dartboard on three out of three chances, and secondly, safety factors had to be considered. Training for accuracy helped eliminate or reduce the chance of stray dart throws that could injure others in the immediate environment. A performance objective, verbal cue, and task analysis appears in Table 7.

Baseline

Initial nonreinforced baselining was carried out to determine preinstruction competency levels. The baseline level for each participant was de-

Table 7. Task analysis for dart toss

Performance Objective: Given a dartboard at standard height and three darts, the participants will strike the dartboard from the standard 8 foot distance, 100% of the time.

Verbal Cue: "(Herman, Roselyn, Robert), throw the darts at the board."

Task Analysis:
1. Stand/sit 8 feet from dartboard.
2. Grasp first dart in dominant hand (tip of dart facing board) using pincer grasp.
3. Bend elbow until forearm is perpendicular to ground.
4. Thrust forearm and hand in forward motion toward board, releasing dart when arm is extended.
5. First dart strikes dartboard.
6. Throw second dart, striking dartboard.
7. Throw third dart, striking dartboard.

rived by giving the verbal cue (i.e., "Herman, Roselyn, Robert, throw the darts at the board."), and recording the steps of the task analysis performed correctly and without assistance. Herman, Roselyn, and Robert, within the multiple baseline design, were baselined on 5, 11, and 14 sessions, respectively. One baseline trial per session was conducted for each participant.

Instruction

Each instructional session consisted of five training trials followed by a nonreinforced probe in which no prompting was offered. The general verbal cue was simply given and the data collected. Instruction began on the next step on the task analysis which had not been performed correctly or without assistance during two consecutive sessions.

A standard cue hierarchy was utilized to teach the dart skills. This entailed initially administering the verbal cue for the step being trained (e.g., step 2—"Herman, grasp the dart.") and socially reinforcing the participant for appropriate behavior. If the verbal prompt did not elicit the desired response, the second stage of the teaching hierarchy was implemented. This included giving the verbal cue and concurrently modeling the correct behavior. The client was then verbally prompted to try again (e.g., "Herman, now you try."). If the targeted behavior was elicited, the player was socially reinforced. Finally, if the participant again failed to perform, the instructor physically prompted the player through the appropriate action, while once again giving the verbal cue. Praise was offered following this hierarchical step. Reinforcement consisted of social praise, pats on back, extra attention, and in one case, edibles.

Training continued for each participant until he or she was capable of performing all seven steps of the task analysis during two consecutive sessions. Generalization probes, in the absence of prompts and reinforcement, were performed in at least two other environments for all participants. Locations for these probes included a friend's apartment, neighborhood darts bar, and another training facility.

Interobserver Agreement

In order to determine reliability for the baseline, instruction, and generalization recordings, an additional observer was utilized on a weekly basis. During reliability checks, the instructor/original data recorder was unaware of the presence of the reliability check. Interobserver reliability averaged 0.98 across the three participants. It was believed that this atypically high rank resulted due to 1) a small number, and 2) easily understood and observed task analyzed steps (three of the steps were easily identified as merely striking or missing the dartboard).

Experimental Design

A multiple-baseline design across subjects was employed. In this design, baseline data were collected across three individuals. After competency levels for each person had stabilized during a one week period (five sessions), instruction commenced on participant 1, Herman. At this time, baseline data collection continued on the other participants. The minimal criterion for his performance that was required in order to implement instruction with participant 2, Roselyn, was 100% increase in task analytic steps performed independently above preinstruction competency levels on 2 consecutive days. The identical procedure was followed for beginning instruction with participant 3, Robert.

Within this evaluation technique a changing-criterion design was utilized for two of the participants. Participant 2 received instruction in which distance from the target and board height were varied. Instruction began at one half distance (4 feet) from the target at the standard board height (5 feet, 8 inches). When this level of performance was obtained (i.e., 100% performance on 2 consecutive days), instruction continued at three-quarters distance (6 feet) at standard board height. Once criterion was met, instruction commenced at standard distance (8 feet). But following 10 sessions without improvement and not striking the dartboard, a modified board height (4 feet, 8 inches) was utilized. Mastery of this height resulted in the board being raised to 5 feet, 2 inches. Standard height (5 feet, 8 inches), along with standard distance was ultimately required for performance to reach the mastery level.

Participant 3 also required instruction using a change in distance criterion. The changing levels of performance were one-half distance, three-quarters distance and standard distance. Board height remained at the normal 5 feet, 8 inches throughout instruction. Participant 1 received instruction to criterion with distance from the dartboard and board height remaining constant.

Results and Discussion

The goal of the leisure skills program was to instruct three severely-profoundly handicapped adults to learn dart skills. Figure 5 illustrates this acquisition within a multiple-baseline design.

For participants 1 and 2, stable baseline rates were obtained at step 2 of the task analysis (i.e., grasping dart using pincer grasp). Subsequently, instruction commenced for these participants at step 3 (i.e., proper positioning of throwing arm). Participant 3 demonstrated a fairly stable baseline at 0-step proficiency. On two occasions, however, Robert was able to stand behind the foul line. During one probe, he exhibited the appropriate dart grasp. This was believed to be due to chance as the behavior returned to 0-rate in subsequent sessions. Therefore, instruction began on step 1 of the task analysis (i.e., stand 8 feet from dart board).

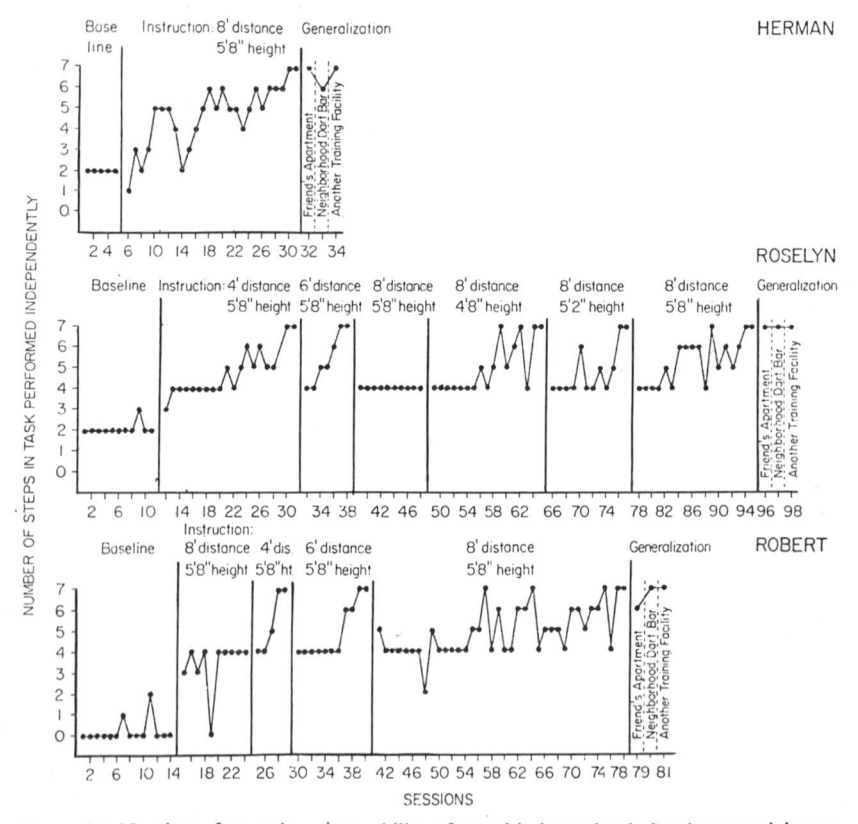

Figure 5. Number of steps in a darts skill performed independently by three participants.

Participant 1, Herman, mastered the darts skills relatively quickly within 26 instructional sessions. In contrast, participants 2 and 3, requiring a changing-criterion method of programming, used a considerably larger number of sessions, 98 and 81 sessions, respectively.

Nonreinforced generalization probes were taken in three different environments outside the home agency. These locations included a friend's apartment, popular neighborhood darts bar, and another training facility within the county. During probes in two of the three sites, 100% criterion was met, and in the third, Herman struck the dartboard on two out of three attempts, certainly an acceptable performance. Roselyn and Robert both achieved acceptable levels in the same three generalization environments.

CONCLUSION

The purpose of this chapter has been to *demonstrate* the assessment techniques, instructional methods, and adaptations discussed in previous chapters. The population focused upon was a severely multihandicapped group of adolescents and young adults. An effort was made to describe how photography, cooking, and dart skills could be implemented. A group home leisure program was also described.

Each of the studies presented daily data and were evaluated in behavioral designs. Behavioral principles were employed for instruction and generalization was programmed in several cases. We hope the programs in this chapter have clarified the concepts and curricula provided within this text.

REFERENCE NOTE

Note 1: Wehman, P., Schleien, S., & Kiernan, J. Age appropriate recreation programs for severely handicapped youth and adults. *Journal of the Association for the Severely Handicapped* (JASH). In press.

REFERENCES

Brown, L. Instructional programs for the trainable level retarded. In L. Mann & D. Sabatin (Eds.), *First annual review of special education*, New York: Grune & Stratton, 1973.

Robinson-Wilson, M. Picture recipe cards as an approach to teaching severely retarded adults to cook. In G. T. Bellamy (Ed.), *Habilitation of the severely and profoundly retarded*. Rehabilitation Research and Training Center, University of Oregon, Eugene, Oregon, 1976, 99–106.

Rombauer, I., & Rombauer-Becker, M. *Joy of cooking*. New York: New American Library, 1964.

Sulzer-Azaroff, B., & Mayer, L. *Applied behavior analysis procedures with children and youth*. New York: Houghton & Mifflin, 1977.

INDEX

Adaptations of leisure skills, 59–86
  in community-based facilities, 77–81
  conditions for, 64–65
  curricula using, 84–85
  guidelines for, 65–67
  historical background for, 60–62
  homemade aids in, 72
  individualized, 66
  leadup activities in, 64, 65, 81–84
  materials and equipment in, 67–73
  and normalization principles, 60, 63
  philosophies concerning, 63–64
  procedures and rules in, 73–76, 161
  programmatic, 65–76
  rationale for, 59–60
  skill sequences in, 76–77
  types of, 67–85
Archery, aids in, 68, 71
Architectural barriers, elimination of, 77–80
Arm movement, as core skill, 94
Arm wrestle, skills in, 172–173
Assessment of leisure skills, 15–33
  and access to materials and events, 30–31
  age-appropriate skills in, 30
  and appropriateness of object manipulation, 21–23
  behavioral variables for, 19–26
  criteria of instruments in, 15–19
  and criteria for skill selection, 26–33
  direction of interactions in, 25–26
  duration of activity in, 20–21
  free play in, 26
  frequency of interactions in, 24–25
  group assessment in, 19
  home environment in, 31–33
  performance level in, 28–29
  physical characteristics in, 29–30
  preference evaluation in, 23–24, 27–28
  and proficiency in skills, 19–20
  task analysis in, 19–20
Attending or focusing, as core skill, 93

Auditory tracking, as core skill, 93
Avocational Activities Inventory, 16

Badminton, skills in, 130–133
Ball games
  baseball, 64, 83
  basketball, 84, 133–135
  handball, 141–143
  kickball, 177–178
  multipurpose ball in, 215–218
  newcomb, 64, 65, 82–83
  softball, 149–152
  tetherball, 181
  volleyball, 64, 65, 75, 82–83, 155–157
Baseball, leadup activities for, 64, 83
Basketball
  leadup activities for, 84
  skills in, 133–135
Behavior
  latency measure of, 23
  modification of, and normalization principle, 10
Behavioral objectives, in leisure education program, 37–38
Behavior variables, for leisure assessment, 19–26
Bicycle use
  aids in, 84
  skills in, 104–106
Billiards or pool
  aids in, 75
  skills in, 126–128
Bingo, skills in, 162–163
Blind persons, adaptations for, 69–71
Blocks, playing with, 198–200
Board games, skills in, 162–172
Bogan's Group Assessment, 16, 19
Book use, skills in, 98–100
Bowling
  adaptations in, 66, 67, 71
  electric bowling game, 125–126
  skills in, 135–138
Bubble-blowing, skills in, 214–215

Bucket and shovel play, skills in, 200–201
Busy Box use, skills in, 202–204

Camera use
  aids in, 77
  case study of training program for, 231–237
  skills in, 113–115
Camping activities, 100–102
Card games, 75–76, 85
  skills in, 190–195
Chaining
  backward, 47
  forward, 47
Checkers, skills in, 163–164
Christmas tree decorating, 106–107
Comic Strips game, 72
Community facilities, accessibility of, 77–81
Comprehensive Evaluation in Recreational Therapy Scale (CERT), 16
Concentration game, skills in, 190–191
Constructive Leisure Activity Survey (CLAS), 16
Cooking
  aids in, 76–77
  case study of training program for, 237–244
  skills in, 102–104
Core skills, 40–41, 45
  and curriculum design, 93–94
Crayon use, skills in, 205
Crossword puzzles, skills for, 164–165
Cue hierarchy, in teaching techniques, 47–49
Curriculum for leisure activities
  activity groupings in, 89–92
  adaptations used in, 84–85
  core skills in, 93–94
  design and format of, 89–95
  field testing of, 95
  skill sequencing in, 92
Cycling
  aids in, 84
  skills in, 104–106

Dance events, skills in, 118–119
Dart-playing
  case study of training program for, 252–259
  modifications in, 84
  skills in, 165–166
Davis' Recreational Director's Observational Report, 16
Deaf-blind persons
  adaptations for, 69–71
  Knox, Hurff & Takata Assessment of, 16
Deinstitutionalization, and recreation programs, 3–4

Easter egg decoration, 107–108
Education program for leisure skills, 37–57
  adaptations of activities in, 59–86
  and assessment of competencies, 15–33
  behavioral objectives in, 37–38
  case studies in
    camera use, 231–237
    cooking skills, 237–244
    dart skills, 252–259
    group home program, 244–252
  core skills in, 40–41, 45, 93–95
  curriculum design and format in, 89–95. *See also* Curriculum for leisure activities
  evaluation of, 55–57
    multiple baseline design in, 57
    pretest-teach-posttest design in, 55–56
    reversal design in, 56
  and evaluation of progress, 41–42
  games in, 161–195
  hobby skills in, 97–128
  and normalization theory, 1–12
  object manipulation skills in, 197–229
  and program development, 37–57
  program implementation in, 231–259
  replicability of, 42
  sequencing of skills in, 39, 42–45
    resources for, 43–44
    steps involved in, 44–45
  sports skills in, 129–160
  task analysis in, 39–42
    and assessment of skills, 19–20
  teaching techniques in, 45–51
  training competencies in, 53–55
  and transfer of training, 11–12, 51–53
Equipment and materials, modifica-

tions in, 67–73
Exercises, for wheelchair patients, 75
Extension of arms or legs, as core skill, 94

Fading, as teaching technique, 46
Families
   and evaluation of home environment, 31–33
   role in transfer of training, 52
Farmer in the Dell, skills in, 184–185
Fishing, skills in, 138–141
Fishing piers, modifications in, 80, 81
Flexion of arms or legs, as core skill, 94
Focusing or attending, as core skill, 93
Follow the leader, skills in, 173–174
Food preparation
   aids in, 76–77
   case study of training program for, 237–244
   skills in, 102–104
Football, skills in, 123–124
Frisbee, skills in, 205–207

Games, 161–195
   board and table games, 162–172
   card games, 190–195
   curriculum model for, 90, 91
   motor games, 172–184
   musical/rhythmical games, 184–190
Gardening activities, and skills in plant care, 116–118
Generalization, and skill development, 11–12, 51–53
Golf, aids in, 79
Grasping, as core skill, 94
Group assessment of leisure skills, 19
Group homes, leisure programming in, 244–252

Handball, skills in, 141–143
Handgripper squeezing, skills in, 207
Hand movement, as core skill, 94
Hand slap, skills in, 174
Head control, as core skill, 93
Hobbies, 97–128
   books and magazines, 98–100
   camping, 100–102
   cooking, 76–77, 102–104, 237–244
   curriculum model for, 90–92

cycling, 84, 104–106
holiday activities, 106–108
musical or rhythmical instruments, 108–110
pet care, 110–113
photography, 77, 113–115, 231–237
plant care, 116–118
spectator events, 118–121
sunbathing, 121–123
table games, 123–128
Hokey-Pokey game, 47, 48
Holiday activities, 106–108
Home environment, evaluation of, 31–33
Hopscotch, skills in, 175–176
Hot potato game, skills in, 186–187
Hula-Hoop use, skills in, 207–210

I Can Curriculum, 16, 18, 19, 84–85
I Doubt It card game, skills in, 191–192
Individual Education Plans (IEP), 6, 9–10
   behavioral objectives in, 37–38
   and curriculum design, 89–95
Individualization of adapting leisure skills, 66
Instruction for leisure skills. *See* Education program
Integration process, concepts in, 6–9
Iowa Leisure Education Program Assessment Form, 16, 19

Jack-in-the-box play, skills in, 210–211
Jacks, skills in, 166–167
Jogging, skills in, 143–144
Joswiak's Leisure Counseling Assessment Instruments, 16
Jumping rope, skills in, 176–177

Kickball, skills in, 177–178
Knox, Hurff & Takata Deaf-Blind Assessment, 16

Latency measure of behavior, 23
Leadup activities, for recreational skills, 64, 65, 81–84
Learning Accomplishment Profile, 28
Leg movement, as core skill, 94

Legislation, on recreational/educational services, 5-6
Leisure Activities Blank (LAB), 16, 18
Leisure education specialists, roles of, 9-12
Leisure Interest Inventory (LII), 17
Leisure Skills Curriculum for Developmentally Disabled Persons (LSCDD), 17, 18, 64, 85
Library use, skills in, 99
Limbo, skills in, 187-188
Linear Model for Individual Treatment in Recreation (LMIT), 17, 18
London Bridge, skills in, 188-189
Lotto, skills in, 167-168

Magazine use, skills in, 98-100
Manipulation of objects. *See* Object manipulation
Marbles, skills for, 168-169, 212-214
Marshmallow roasting, skills in, 100
Materials and equipment, modifications in, 67-73
Medical model of human services, objections to, 10
Minimum Objective System (MOS), 17, 18, 28
Mirenda Leisure Interest Finder, 17, 19
Modeled behavior, as teaching technique, 46
Modified activities. *See* Adaptations of leisure skills
Motor games, skills in, 172-184
Movie attendance, skills in, 118
Musical chairs, skills in, 189-190
Musical games, skills in, 184-190
Musical instruments, use of, 108-110, 185-186

Newcomb, as modification of volleyball, 64, 65, 82-83
Normalization of disabled persons, 1-12
  and adaptation of activities, 60, 63
  and behavior modification, 10
  and concepts of integration process, 6-9
  cooperative approach to, 9
  historical aspects of, 2-3
  individualized programs in, 6, 9-10
  legislative acts on, 5-6
  and leisure time activities, 2, 4-5
  and research in recreation studies, 4-5
  and roles of leisure education specialists, 9-12
  and trends in community services, 3-4

Object manipulation, 197-229
  appropriateness of, 21-23
  blocks in, 198-200
  crayons in, 205
  curriculum model for, 90, 91
  frisbee in, 205-207
  handgripper in, 207
  Hula-Hoop in, 207-210
  jack-in-the-box in, 210-211
  marbles in, 212-214
  Mr. Bubble in, 214-215
  multipurpose ball in, 215-218
  scissors in, 218-220
  Slinky in, 220-222
  telephone in, 222-227
  vending machines in, 227-229
Old Maid game, skills in, 192-193
Parachute play, skills in, 178-179
Parents. *See* Families
Personnel for leisure education, roles of, 9-12
Pet care, skills in, 110-113
Photography
  aids in, 77
  case study of training program for, 231-237
  skills in, 113-115
Physical characteristics, assessment of, 29-30
Physical recreation. *See* Sports
Pinball, skills in, 124-125, 169-170
Ping pong
  aids in, 71
  skills in, 170-171
Plant care, skills in, 116-118
Play behavior, assessment of, 26
Playground equipment
  modifications of, 82
  skills involved in use of, 144-148
Pool and billiards

aids in, 75
skills in, 126–128
Preferences in leisure activities, evaluation of, 23–24, 27–28
Proficiency in leisure skills, evaluation of, 19–20
Progress in leisure education, evaluation of, 41–42
Prompting, as teaching technique, 46
Public buildings, accessibility of, 77–81

Record player use, skills in, 119–120
Recreation Therapy Assessment, 17
Reinforcement, in education program, 49–51
  amount of, 50–51
  effectiveness of, 49–50
  schedule of, 51
  timing of, 50
Reinforcers
  naturally occurring, 51–52
  sampling of, 49
Rhythmical games, skills in, 184–190
Rhythmical instruments, use of, 108–110, 185–186
Rules and regulations for games, modifications in, 73–76, 161

Sand play, activities in, 200–202
Scissors use
  adaptations in, 69–71
  skills in, 218–220
See-saw play, skills in, 144–145
Self-Leisure Interest Profile (SLIP), 17
Sequencing of skills. *See* Skill sequences
Sewing
  aids in, 71, 72–73
  leadup activities for, 84
Shaping of behavior, 46–47
Shuffleboard, skills in, 148–149
Simon Says game, skills in, 179–180
Sitting unsupported, as core skill, 94
Skill sequences in education program, 39, 42–45
  and curriculum design, 92
  modifications in, 76–77
Slap Jack game, skills in, 193–194
Sledding, skills in, 159–160

Sleeping bag use, skills in, 101
Sliding board play, skills in, 145–147
Slinky use, skills in, 220–222
Snowball making, skills in, 158–159
Social interactions
  direction of, 25–26
  frequency of, 24–25
Softball, skills in, 149–152
Sonoma County Organization for the Retarded Assessment System (SCOR), 17, 18
Specialists in leisure education, roles of, 9–12
Spectator events, skills in, 118–121
Sports programs, 129–160. *See also* Ball games
  adaptations in, 61–62
  badminton, 130–133
  basketball, 84, 133–135
  bowling, 66, 67, 71, 135–138
  curriculum model for, 91, 92
  fishing, 80, 81, 138–141
  handball, 141–143
  jogging, 143–144
  and playground equipment, 82, 144–148
  shuffleboard, 148–149
  softball, 149–152
  swimming, 72, 81, 152–155
  volleyball, 64, 65, 75, 82–83, 155–157
  weightlifting, 72, 157–158
  in winter, 158–160
Standing unsupported, as core skill, 41, 94
State of Ohio Curriculum Guide for Moderately Mentally Retarded Learners, 17, 19
Sunbathing, skills in, 121–123
Swimming
  aids in, 72, 81
  skills in, 152–155
  and sunbathing skills, 121–123
Swing play, skills in, 147–148

Table games
  skills in, 123–128, 162–172
  for wheelchair users, 79
Tag games, skills in, 180–181
Task analysis
  in assessment of leisure skills, 19–20

Task analysis—*continued*
  and leisure education, 39–42
Teaching techniques, in education program for leisure skills, 45–51
  cue hierarchy in, 47–49
  fading in, 46
  modeling in, 46
  prompting in, 46
  reinforcement in, 49–51
  shaping and chaining in, 46–47
  and trainer competencies, 53–55
Telephone use
  aids in, 62, 68, 78–79, 81
  leadup activities for, 83
  skills in, 222–227
Television use, skills in, 94, 121
Tennis
  aids in, 65, 72, 85
  leadup activities for, 65, 84
Tetherball, skills in, 181
Tic-tac-toe, skills for, 171–172
Toward Competency: A Guide for Individualized Instruction, 17
Toy play. *See* Object manipulation
Transfer of training, 11–12, 51–53
  and alterations in reinforcement variables, 52
  family role in, 52
  practical suggestions for, 53
  and varying stimulus conditions, 52–53
Tug of war, skills in, 182–183
Twister game, skills in, 183–184

Vending machine use
  aids in, 82
  skills in, 227–229
Vineland Social Maturity Scale, 17, 18
Visual tracking, as core skill, 93
Volleyball
  aids in, 75
  leadup activities for, 64, 65, 82–83
  skills in, 155–157

War card games, skills in, 194–195
Water fountains, modifications of, 82
Weightlifting
  aids in, 72
  skills in, 157–158
Wheelchair users
  adaptations for, 78–80
  sports programs for, 61, 73
Winter sports, skills in, 158–160
Wrestling, arm, skills in, 172–173